ARTHUR S. KEATS L[...]
TEXAS HEART INSTITUTE

P9-DDI-978

PHARMACOLOGIC MANAGEMENT OF PERIOPERATIVE BLEEDING

Andrew S. Wechsler, MD

Pharmacologic Management of Perioperative Bleeding

Pharmacologic Management of Perioperative Bleeding

Andrew S. Wechsler, MD
Stuart McGuire Professor and Chairman
Department of Surgery
Medical College of Virginia
Virginia Commonwealth University
Richmond, Virginia

CME Network, Publishing/Southampton, New York

Publisher:	Carol Lieberman CME Network 41 Barkers Island Road Southampton, NY 11968 (516) 283-7959 FAX (516) 283-4932
Medical Editors:	Barbara Royston Jack Adler
Managing Editor:	Mary Anne Gray
Editor:	Doris F. Innis
Layout and Design:	Thomas Gabrielli

Pharmacologic Management of Perioperative Bleeding

© 1996 by CME Network. All rights reserved. No part of this book may be reproduced, reused, republished, or transmitted in any form or by any means without written permission of the publisher.

Printed in the United States of America

Library of Congress Catalog Card Number: 96-83935

Pharmacologic Management of Perioperative Bleeding

Edited by Andrew S. Wechsler, MD

Acknowledgment

This book represents the proceedings of a symposium—Pharmacologic Management of Perioperative Bleeding—held February 14-15, 1995, in Orlando, Florida. It was made possible by an unrestricted educational grant from Bayer Corporation, Pharmaceutical Division.

CONTENTS

WORKSHOP I:
BLOOD CONSERVATION IN ORTHOPEDIC SURGERY

WORKSHOP II:
BLOOD CONSERVATION IN TRANSPLANT SURGERY

WORKSHOP III:
NEW ASPECTS OF HEMOSTATIC TRANSFUSION

Contributors

Wolf O. Bechstein, MD
Department of Surgery, Vichow Clinic, Humboldt University,
Berlin, Germany

Marcus E. Carr Jr, MD, PhD
Associate Professor of Medicine/Pathology, Medical College of Virginia
Richmond, Virginia, USA

Ola E. Dahl, MD
Research Forum, Department of Orthopaedics, Ullevaal University Hospital,
Oslo, Norway

Anthony M. D'Alessandro, MD
Associate Professor of Surgery, Transplant Service, University of Wisconsin
Medical School, Madison, Wisconsin, USA

Jawed Fareed, PhD
Professor of Pathology and Pharmacology, Director, Hemostasis and
Thrombosis Research Laboratories, Loyola University Chicago, Maywood,
Illinois, USA

Robert A. Fisher, MD
Assistant Professor, Surgery and Pediatrics, Director of Liver Transplant
Program, Medical College of Virginia, Richmond, Virginia, USA

Keith A.A. Fox, MB, ChB, FRCP
Duke of Edinburgh Professor of Cardiology and Head of Department,
Cardiovascular Research Unit, Edinburgh, United Kingdom

Lawrence T. Goodnough, MD
Department of Pathology and Medicine, Washington University School of
Medicine, St. Louis, Missouri, USA

Sylvia Haas, MD
Professor of Medicine, Institute for Experimental Surgery, Technical
University, Munich, Germany

Laurence A. Harker, MD
Blomeyer Professor of Medicine, Director of the Division of Hematology-
Oncology, Emory University, Atlanta, Georgia, USA

Gary Hartstein, MD
Assistant Professor of Anesthesiology, University Hospital of Liege, Liege,
Belgium

Valluvan Jeevanandam, MD
Assistant Professor of Surgery, Surgical Director, Heart Failure and
Transplant Program, Temple University, Philadelphia, Pennsylvania, USA

Harvey G. Klein, MD
Chief, Department of Transfusion Medicine, National Institutes of Health,
Bethesda, Maryland, USA

Robert Mervyn Letts, MD, FRCP
Head, Department of Surgery, Children's Hospital of Eastern Ontario
University of Ottawa, Ottawa, Ontario, Canada

J. Lance Lichtor, MD
Professor of Anesthesia and Critical Care, University of Chicago,
Chicago, Illinois, USA

Colin Longstaff, PhD
National Institute for Biological Standards and Control, South Mimms, Hertfordshire, England

He Lu, MD
Hopital Saint Louis INSERM U 353, Paris, France

John M. Murkin, MD, FRCPC
Professor, Department of Anaesthesia, University Hospital, University of Western Ontario, London, Ontario, Canada

Michael G. Neuwirth, MD
Hospital for Joint Diseases Orthopaedic Institute, New York, New York, USA

Roque Pifarré, MD
Professor and Chairman Department of Thoracic and Cardiovascular Surgery, Loyola University of Chicago Stritch School of Medicine, Maywood, Illinois, USA

Colin R.M. Prentice, MD, FRCP
Professor of Medicine, Leeds General Infirmary, Leeds, England

Andrew D. Rosenberg, MD
Vice-Chairman, Department of Anesthesiology, Hospital for Joint Diseases Orthopaedic Institute, New York, New York, USA

David Royston, MD, FFARCS
Consultant in Cardiothoracic Anesthesia, Harefield Hospital, Harefield, Middlesex, England

Bradford S. Schwartz, MD
Section of Hematology, Department of Medicine, University of Wisconsin, Chief of Hematology, Wm. A. Middleton Veterans Affairs Medical Center, Madison, Wisconsin, USA

Michael Sobel, MD
Chief, Vascular Surgery Service, Professor of Surgery, H.H. McGuire Veterans Affairs Medical Center, Medical College of Virginia, Richmond, Virginia, USA

Claudine Soria, PhD, Professor
Laboratoire d'Hematologie, Hopital Lariboisiere, Paris. France

Jeannette Soria, PhD, Professor
Laboratoiré Sainte Marie, Hôtel Dieu, Paris. France

James H. Southard, PhD
Professor of Surgery, University of Wisconsin Medical School, Madison, Wisconsin, USA

Jeanine M. Walenga, PhD
Associate Professor, Hemostasis and Thrombosis Research Laboratories Loyola University Chicago, Maywood, Illinois, USA

Andrew S. Wechsler, MD
Stuart McGuire Professor and Chairman, Department of Surgery, Medical College of Virginia, Virginia Commonwealth University, Richmond, Virginia, USA

R. Patrick Wood, MD
Associate Professor, Chief, Liver Transplant Program, University of Texas Medical School, Houston, Texas, USA

Foreword

This book constitutes the proceedings of a symposium entitled Pharmacologic Management of Perioperative Bleeding. It addresses patient risk management during surgery, highlighting pharmacologic concerns of surgeons, orthopedists, hematologists, and anesthesiologists.

The term risk management is heard in all areas of medicine, and quality of patient care and its associated costs are of paramount concern to practitioners. This volume will enable the user to:

- better understand the etiology of perioperative bleeding and hemostatic dysfunction

- identify parameters of the patient at risk in orthopedic, cardiac, and transplant dysfunction

- assess patient need for transfusion or pharmacologic intervention

- define available modalities for pharmacologic intervention

- utilize diagnostic parameters to treat specific perioperative abnormal coagulation states

Both the symposium and this book were funded under an unrestricted educational grant from the Bayer Corporation, Pharmaceutical Division. For the past 4 years, Bayer has supported risk management symposia in conjunction with the Society of Thoracic Surgeons and Society of Cardiovascular Anesthesiologists Annual Meetings. These programs have addressed the most up-to-date trends in journals. In the present case, the enormity of the project and the organizers' desire to publish in book form resulted in this publication.

Ellison C. Pierce Jr, MD
Chairman Emeritus
Department of Anaesthesia
New England Deaconess Hospital
Boston, Massachusetts
Scientific Director,
Pharmacologic Management of Perioperative Bleeding

PREFACE

Surgeons generally have been more apt to create bleeding than adept at stopping it. Were that not the case, no one would ever die or develop complications as a consequence of bleeding difficulties. That should be reason enough to be concerned about the problem of perioperative hemostasis, but recent emphasis on the costs of health care provides additional reason. The cost of running an operating room ranges from $20 to $80 a minute, depending on the institution, so any extra time required to stop bleeding substantially increases the cost of a patient's operating room and hospital stays.

Also, we have begun to increasingly appreciate the deleterious consequences of transfusing blood and blood products, particularly in quantity. These consequences include patient morbidity, expanded ICU and hospital stays, increased complexity of patient ICU management, and heightened potential for complications. Moreover, they add to the difficulty of managing high-risk cases in today's highly competitive medical-market environment in which the focus is on streamlining the management of surgical patients. So reasons for controlling this very important risk factor for operative outcomes are both medical and pragmatic.

The action of pharmacologic agents in improving hemostasis in at-risk groups of patients undergoing major surgery was a major component of the Pharmacologic Management of Perioperative Bleeding conference, with particular emphasis placed on the role of serine protease inhibitors and on their efficacy and possible mechanism of action.

This book represents the consensus derived from the clinical and research experiences reported by the specialty groups of invited experts and participants at the conference. The expectation is that this consensus will lead the way to development of improved methods of further reducing perioperative bleeding and the need for donor-blood transfusion.

Andrew S. Wechsler, MD

ix

Risks of Perioperative Transfusion: The Transfusion Trigger

Harvey G. Klein, MD

The concept of a transfusion trigger probably has its roots in a 1942 article in *Clinical Anesthesia*[1] in which Lundy et al stated: "When the concentration of hemoglobin is less than 10 grams per 100 cc of whole blood, it is wise to transfuse before operation." However, it is very difficult, if not impossible, to find any physiologic basis for this conclusion, and the concept has been largely abandoned. The conclusions of a 1988 National Institutes of Health (NIH) consensus conference on perioperative transfusion[2] serve as our guide to practice today, even though they, too, are supported by few scientific data. This panel of well-known and highly regarded experts concluded that no scientific evidence supports the 10/30 rule; no single measurement can replace good clinical judgment; mild to moderate anemia does not contribute to perioperative morbidity; and allogeneic transfusion carries a number of risks.

TRANSFUSION RISKS

The risks associated with the transfusion of units of red cells in the United States in 1996 are shown in Table l.

Table 1. Estimated Risks of Transfusion per Unit in the United States (1996)	
Minor allergic reactions	1:100
Viral hepatitis	1:50,000
Hemolytic transfusion reaction	1:6000
Fatal hemolytic reaction	1:600,000
HIV infection	1:420,000*
HTLV-I/II infection	1:200,000
Bacterial infection (platelets)	1:2500
Acute lung injury	1:500,000
Anaphylactic shock	1:500,000
Graft-versus-host disease	Rare
Immunosuppression	?

*1:340,000 with additional 20% exclusion for other markers.
HIV, Human immunodeficiency virus; HTLV-I, human T-cell lymphotropic virus type 1.

There is about a 1% risk of minor allergic reactions, which include chills, fever, and hives. These may be annoying to patients and physicians, but the cost and inconvenience of workup aside, not very problematic. The risk of viral hepatitis today is about 1 case in every 50,000 units of transfused blood. With use of the third-generation hepatitis C screening test, licensed in Europe but not in the United States, the risk is probably only l in 60,000 to 80,000 units of blood transfused. Based on the prevalence of hepatitis in the United States, the calculated "window period" of screening test negativity, the transmissibility by transfusion, and the effectiveness of other screening procedures, some researchers have calculated the risk to be as low as 1 infection in 100,000 units. Hemolytic transfusion reactions occur with about 1 in every 6000 units; fatal reactions occur with about 1 in every 600,000 units transfused.

The risk of contracting the human immunodeficiency virus (HIV) is a major concern of the American public. In actuality, this is currently a small problem in the United States. If the risk is calculated by using the period between when a prospective donor is infected and when his test becomes positive and his blood donation thus rejected, the estimated prevalence of HIV in normal donors, and the elimination of donors because of screening tests, the estimated risk is about 1 unit of infectious blood in every 420,000 units of blood transfused. This translates into, at most, 100 cases of infection caused by transfused blood a year; about half of these patients will not live long enough to develop clinical evidence of the acquired immunodeficiency syndrome (AIDS). In addition, a further safeguard in the form of a test for HIV antigen has recently been added to the screening process.

Other infection risks involve human T-cell lymphotropic virus type I (HTLV-I) and type II, other retroviruses, and bacterial infection. Bacterial infection of blood components may be largely underrecognized. In platelets, which are stored at room temperature, as many as 1 unit in every 2500 appears to be infected when cultured. However, we rarely see severe problems due to bacterial infection in patients after platelet transfusion, perhaps because many of these patients are on antibiotics or because the culture of a platelet bag cannot be equated with patient infections for other reasons. It is possible that this complication goes unrecognized or is underreported. Only a handful of bacterial infections related to red cells stored at refrigerated temperature are reported each year.

Acute lung injury, which certainly can occur after surgical procedures, and anaphylactic shock occurs very rarely. Graft-versus-host disease (GVHD) resulting from immunocompetent lymphocytes given to a somewhat immunosuppressed patient is very rare but almost invariably fatal. Nevertheless, these are well-recognized complications of allogeneic blood.

Ironically, there is now considerable public concern about the safety of our blood supply, whereas in the past there was practically none. In fact, our blood supply has become dramatically safer over the last 30 years. As noted above, with our current systems of identification of donor and recipient, the risk of a fatal acute transfusion reaction now is about 1 in 600,000. In contrast, in 1942 Kilduffe and Debakey reported a rate of about 1 in 1000 and other studies reported a similar range.[3] Studies done at the NIH in the 1960s showed an incidence of active hepatitis infection of about 30% after open heart surgery. With the introduction of all volunteer blood, reduction in the units transfused per case, additional screening tests and various procedures designed specifically to decrease the risk of HIV, the risk of incurring hepatitis at the NIH dropped dramatically; only one case has been found in the last 500 patients followed prospectively. And, despite the common attribution of hepatitis C in a patient to a transfusion, at most only 6% of cases of hepatitis C in the United States are caused by blood transfusion.[4] Of the remaining cases, about 40% are due to IV drug use, probably somewhat less than 6% to sexual exposure, and a very small number are caused by household or occupational exposure. The causes of 40% of cases remain unknown, but we do know they are not the consequence of blood transfusion.

Similarly, transfusion-transmitted HIV infection is now negligible. The peak of HIV infection as a function of either first date or last date of transfusion was reached in 1984 or 1985. Almost no transfusion-transmitted AIDS is seen after the introduction of measures to remove high-risk donors and the availability of a screening test. There have been only 35 cases of AIDS related to transfusion since 1985. Of course, given the long incubation period of HIV, it is possible that the true number of cases may be twice or even three times that; nevertheless, this possible annual incidence of, at most, less than 100 cases occurred with about 14 million units of blood and blood components being transfused every year in the United States.

Other Infectious Agents

Besides hepatitis A, B, C, and D, HIV-l and 2, HTLV-I and II, and bacteria (Table 2), there are other infectious agents that may be transmitted by blood. For example, a virus recently designated hepatitis G virus (HGV), which is probably the cause of the residual non-A, non-B hepatitis, is transmitted by blood and poses a small risk of hepatitis. Other viruses we are aware of include cytomegalovirus (CMV), the Epstein-Barr virus, and parvovirus Bl9. Although we know of several retroviruses, there are undoubtedly others posing a potential threat that cannot be detected by current tests. There also may be other new or emerging agents that remain to be identified. For example, some investigators have raised concerns about an agent responsible for Creutzfeldt-Jakob disease (CJD) as a possible transfusion-transmissible agent.[5]

Table 2. Infectious Agents Transmitted by Transfusion

Viruses	Parasites
Hepatitis A, B, C, D	Plasmodia
HIV-1,2	*Babesia microti*
HTLV-I,II	*Trypanosoma cruzi*
Cytomegalovirus	*Toxoplasma gondii*
Epstein-Barr virus	*Leishmania donovani*
Parvovirus B19	
Spirochetes	**Bacteria**
	Staphylococcus
Treponema pallidum	Salmonella
Borrelia burgdorferi	Yersinia enterocolitica

HIV, Human immunodeficiency virus; HTLV-I, human T-cell lymphotropic virus type 1.

Spirochetes can be transmitted by blood, although this rarely occurs. Certainly the agent that causes Lyme disease in theory could be transmitted by blood, although such transmission has never been described.

Worldwide, parasites such as malaria are by far the major problem. Only one or two cases a year are identified in the United States. Chagas's disease, problematic in the southern United States, California, and Texas, is an increasing worry; a screening test is now being tested experimentally.[6]

There are agents that we do not think about because they are not yet present in the United States, although they may be problematic elsewhere. What I describe as the Leishmania paradigm is instructive: An unusual syndrome developed among some of the half million young Americans sent to the Persian Gulf in 1991. It was found that 22 of these military personnel were infected with *Leishmania tropica*. Although nothing was known about this species, it was known that the related organism *L. donovani* has a parasitemic phase and can be transmitted by blood. On that basis, all half million servicepersons, all potential blood donors, were removed from the blood-donor pool for a year. The lesson here is that as we send Americans around the globe, we will recognize new blood-borne agents; consequently, our donor pool could be significantly and immediately reduced.

ALLOGENEIC TRANSFUSIONS AND THE IMMUNE RESPONSE

There is laboratory evidence that allogeneic transfusions can alter the immune response, posing a potential risk of immune suppression.[7] Laboratory studies show that patients who have received allogeneic blood transfusions show development of FcR-blocking factors, decreased numbers of lymphocytes and helpers, and increased numbers of suppressors, all of which can persist for months after transfusion. Other findings include an increased number of "activated" lymphocytes and down-regulation of antigen-presenting cells. Other abnormalities have been recognized in both B and T cells.

There is much to suggest that these immunomodulating effects of allogeneic transfusions are clinically important. We know that there is improved organ allograft survival, certainly in heart or kidney transplants, after blood transfusion. There are data suggesting that there may be recurrence or decreased survival in patients with malignancies who receive blood during their operative procedures.[8] There may be increased susceptibility to infection after allogeneic blood transfusions, particularly in the perioperative setting.[9] There are some data suggesting that allogeneic blood may prevent recurrent spontaneous abortion by immunosuppressing the mother.[10] There are also some data suggesting that allogeneic blood can suppress inflammatory disease; patients with Crohn's disease who have had bowel resection with allogeneic transfusion seem to have less recurrence and longer recurrence-free survival than those who have not.[11] Laboratory culture data suggest that allogeneic blood reactivates latent viruses.[12] And finally, we know that immunoactive lymphocytes in blood transfusions can cause a clearly immune-mediated and fatal GVHD.[13]

The earliest data suggesting that allogeneic blood had an immunosuppressive effect were published in 1978. Opelz et al[14] reported that patients receiving transplants of cadaver kidneys had better graft survival if they had received allogeneic blood, with survival directly related in dose-response fashion to the amount of allogeneic blood they had received. Although these retrospective data were highly controversial at the time, the effect they indicated was subsequently confirmed. The effect appears much less important in this era of cyclosporine and other potent drug-induced immuosuppression regimens. Nevertheless, Lagaaij et al[15] reported in 1989 that in patients receiving heart or kidney transplants, whether from cadavers or, in the case of kidneys, from a living relative, graft survival improved significantly when there was at least one shared HLA class 2 haplotype between the unit of transfused blood and the recipient.

An immunosuppressive effect by blood transfusion on the recurrence of cancer in patients operated on for their malignancy was first postulated in 1981.[16] Subsequently, about 30 papers have been published specifically on this effect in patients with colorectal carcinoma. In the majority of these retrospective studies, patients who received blood transfusions had decreased survival or decreased tumor-free survival compared with those who did not.

The data are striking, despite the very legitimate critique that patients who received the most blood were those with the most severe disease or the widest spread of cancer.

A number of prospective studies have attempted to address this issue. Four such studies are listed in Table 3. Ness et al[17] studied 315 consecutive prostatectomies for prostate cancer performed at Johns Hopkins, comparing outcomes in patients receiving autologous or allogeneic blood. They found no difference in survival or recurrence of cancer between the two groups. However, the design for this study did not permit randomization. A recently published study by Heiss et al[18] randomized 120 patients undergoing surgery for colorectal carcinoma to receive 2 units of either autologous or allogeneic blood. The patients randomized to receive autologous blood showed significantly better survival than those in the allogeneic blood group. However, this study can be criticized because a high percentage of patients who received autologous blood also received allogeneic blood, and many patients who were in the allogeneic arm of the study received no blood at all.

Table 3. Blood Transfusion and Cancer Recurrence; Prospective Studies

Study	Design	Subjects	Control	Results
Ness et al., 1992	PNR	315 Prostate CA	Autologous	NS
Heiss et al., 1992	PR	120/520 Colorectal	Autologous	$P<.05$
Busch et al., 1993	PR	475 Colorectal	Autologous	NS
Houbiers, et al, 1994	PR	871/1108 Colorectal	Leukocyte-depleted	NS

PNR, prospective nonrandomized; PR, prospective randomized; CA, cancer; NS, not significant.

A very similar study of colorectal carcinoma outcomes was conducted in 14 centers in the Netherlands and one in the United Kingdom, using 2 units of autologous blood as the control.[19] This study found no difference in outcomes between the two groups. A comparison of outcomes in transfused patients with outcomes in nontransfused patients showed that the transfused patients clearly did worse; however, patients had not been randomized on this basis.

Finally, in a similar study, patients undergoing curative colorectal surgery in the Netherlands received either leukocyte-depleted or non-leukocyte-depleted blood.[20] There was no difference between the two groups in cancer recurrence or total survival. However, those patients who received any transfusion, whether leukocyte-depleted or not, had earlier recurrence and decreased survival compared with patients who had received no transfusion, although patients were not randomized on this basis. It is certainly possible that the patients who received transfusions were sicker or required more extensive surgery than those who did not. Thus, the issue of whether allogeneic blood has an immunosuppressive effect is an open and interesting, if controversial, area.

A related interesting but controversial area is that of the immunomodulation of the immune response by allogeneic transfusion and its possible relationship to infection. There are now about 25 reported retrospective studies that have explored this question, but they are poorly controlled for a variety of reasons: It is difficult to arrive at a good definition of infection from chart reviews; differences between surgeons in practice and technique may be more crucial to outcomes than the distinction between allogeneic and autologous blood; patients receiving autologous blood may be healthier than those receiving allogeneic blood; and if patients receiving autologous blood really do have more infections than those who receive no transfusion, it may be because they are sicker to begin with, so that transfusion is just a surrogate marker.

In 17 of the 19 studies I have reviewed, transfusion proved to be a significant predictor of postoperative infection. In 12 of these 17 studies, transfusion was the single best predictor of infection. With multivariate analysis, factors that predict transfusion (eg, hematocrit, blood loss, duration of surgery) were not significant predictors of postoperative infection but allogeneic transfusion was. In the few studies that used autologous blood as a control, autologous transfusion of comparable amount resulted in fewer postoperative infections.

There are now five prospective randomized studies of the effect of allogeneic blood on infection rates in different kinds of surgical procedures (Table 4); four of the five used either leukocyte-depleted or autologous blood as controls. In four of the studies, a statistically significant relationship between perioperative infections and allogeneic blood is shown.[19,21,22]

Table 4. Transfusion and Postoperative Infection; Prospective Studies

Study	Design	Subjects	Control	Results
Braga et al, 1992	PNR	285 Gastric colon, pancreas	None	$P<.05$
Jensen et al, 1992	PR	197 Colorectal	Leukocyte-depleted	$P<.01$
Heiss et al, 1993	PR	120/520 Colorectal	Autologous	$P<.05$
Busch et al, 1993	PR	475 Colorectal	Autologous	NS
Houbiers, et al, 1994	PR	871/1108 Colorectal	Leukocyte-depleted	$P<.001$

PNR, prospective nonrandomized; PR, prospective randomized; NS, not significant.

Treatment of Recurrent Spontaneous Abortion With Allogeneic Blood
Mowbray et al[10] conducted a paired, sequential, double-blind trial to look at spontaneous abortion as an immune-mediated entity that might be prevented by immunosuppression with allogeneic blood. Couples were randomized with lymphocytes collected from 1 unit of whole blood either from the husband (allogeneic transfusion) or from the wife as an autologous control. Three milliliter cell suspensions were infused either intravenously or subcutaneously. Serial testing for antipaternal antibodies was performed. Among the women who received their husbands' lymphocytes, 17 live births and 5 abortions occurred in the next 22 pregnancies. Among the women who re-

ceived their own lymphocytes, only 10 live births and 17 abortions occurred in 27 pregnancies. The study was stopped early because of the highly statistically significant difference in outcomes between the two groups that suggested that there was something about allogeneic lymphocytes that allowed women with multiple spontaneous abortions to carry their next pregnancy to term.

Transfusion-Related Immunomodulation and AIDS
Four studies have indicated that individuals who have AIDS and receive blood transfusions have a worse clinical course, suggesting an immunosuppressive effect by allogeneic transfusion. Whyte et al[23] found that among patients at high risk for AIDS, survival was significantly shorter for transfused patients. Ward et al[24] found that the progression of AIDS was more rapid in transfusion recipients compared with controls. Vamvakas and Kaplan[25] found decreased survival associated with transfusions. Sloand et al[26] showed increased frequency of CMV, wasting, and bacterial infection among AIDS patients who received transfusion.

It has long been known that the culturing of HIV-infected cells with phytohemagglutinin (PHA) results in an increased amount of HIV-related antigen in the supernatant in a dose-response mode. Busch et al[12] showed that if allogeneic donor mononuclear cells are cocultured with lymphocytes from a patient with HIV, the allogeneic cells appear to up-regulate latent virus in the HIV-infected cells, again with a dose-related response. The effect is apparent whether the coculturing is done only with granulocytes, monocytes, or lymphocytes or with unfractionated cells. However, white cell-free plasma, platelets, or red blood cells cause no stimulation of HIV. Thus it appears that white cells, which are present in most units of blood even though not seen, can stimulate latent HIV infections.

Allogeneic Blood and Tumor Growth
Speir et al[27] showed that patients undergoing coronary angioplasty developed immediate restenosis that was related to smooth-muscle cell growth in 25% to 40% of cases. They found that p-53 tumor suppressor proteins, one gene product that suppresses tumor growth in normal individuals, were present in the smooth-muscle cells that seemed to be growing out of control, almost like a benign neoplasm. Smooth muscle that was infected with CMV produced an early protein (lE-84) that increased in accordance with the p-53 gene product. This CMV early immediate protein bound to the p-53 gene product, abolishing its ability to transactivate a reporter gene, thus neutralizing the p-53 gene product. In the light of these findings, it should be remembered that allogeneic blood transfusion can up-regulate and activate latent CMV, allowing it to produce the kinds of proteins that may neutralize the p-53 gene product and thus facilitate uncontrolled growth.

CAUSES OF THE TRANSFUSION EFFECT
Possible causes of the transfusion effect include development of a suppressor cell network, anti-idiotype antibody formation, clonal deletion, macrophage paralysis, or the transmission and up-regulation of infectious agents. Collection/storage contaminants (eg, DEHP) may be involved. All of the above, and other factors as well, may be involved.

GENERAL MANAGEMENT PRINCIPLES
In the absence of any hard and fast transfusion trigger, certain general management principles provide a sound approach to transfusion. The physician should determine the nature of the patient's anemia, determine the goals of

transfusion, consider alternative therapies, anticipate the need for autologous transfusion, and discuss risks and benefits with the patient. And, despite all the potential risks associated with blood transfusions discussed above, it is well to remember Woody Allen's insightful rejoinder: "Blood is still the best possible thing to have in our veins."

References

1. Lundy JS. Clinical Anesthesia: *Manual of Clinical Anesthesiology.* WB Saunders: Philadelphia, Pa. 1942.

2. NIH Consensus Conference. Perioperative red blood cell transfusion. *JAMA* 1988;260:2700-2703.

3. Kilduffe RA, Debakey M. *The Blood Bank and the Technique and Therapeutics of Transfusion.* St. Louis, Mo: Mosby;1942.

4. Alter MJ, Hadler SC, Judson FN, et al. Risk factors for acute non A, non B hepatitis in the United States and association with hepatitis C virus infection. *JAMA* 1990;264:2231-2235.

5. Manuelidis EE, Kim JH, Mevicangos JR, Manuelidis L. Transmission to animals of Creutzfeldt-Jakob disease from human blood. *Lancet* 1985;ii:896-897.

6. Kirchhoff LV. Is Trypanosoma Cruzi a new threat to our blood supply? *Ann InternMed* 1989;iii:773-775.

7. Brunson, ME, Alexander JW: Mechanisms of transfusion induced immunosuppression. *Transfusion* 1990;30:651-658.

8. Blumberg N, Heal JM. Transfusion and host defenses against cancer recurrence and infection. *Transfusion* 1988;29:236-245.

9. Murphy P, Heal JM, Blumberg N. Infection or suspected infection after hip replacement surgery with autologous or homologous blood transfusions. *Transfusion* 1991;31:212-217.

10. Mowbray JF, Lidell H, Underwood JL, et al. Controlled trial of treatment of recurrent spontaneous abortion by immunization with paternal cells. *Lancet* 1985;2:941-943.

11. Williams JG, Hughes LE. Effect of perioperative blood transfusion on recurrence of Crohn's disease. *Lancet* 1989;2:1524. Letter.

12 Busch MP, Lee TH, Heitman J. Allogeneic lymphocytes but not therapeutic blood elements induce reactivation and dissemination of latent HIV-1: implications for transfusion support of infected patients. *Blood* 1992;83:2128-2133.

13 Anderson KC, Weinstein H. Transfusion-associated graft-versus-host disease. *N Engl J Med* 1990;323:315-321.

14 Opelz G, Terasaki PI. Improvement of kidney-graft survivial with increased numbers of blood transfusions. *N Engl J Med* 1978;299:799-803.

15 Lagaaij EL, Hennemann IPH, Ruigrok M, et al. Effect of one-HLA-Dr-antigen-matched and completely HLA-Dr mismatched blood transfusion on survival of heart and kidney allografts. *N Engl J Med* 1989;321:701-705.

16 Burrows L, Tartar P. Effect of blood transfusions on colonic malignancy recurrent rate. *Lancet* 1982;2:662. Letter.

17 Ness PM, Walsh PC, Zahurak M, et al. Prostate cancer recurrence in radical surgery patients receiving autologous or homologous blood. *Transfusion* 1992;32:31-36.

18 Heiss MM, Jauch KW, Delanoff CH, et al. Blood transfusion modulated tumor recurrence: a randomized study of autologous versus homologous blood transfusion in colorectal cancer. *Proc Annu Meet AM Soc Clin Oncol* 1992;11:172. Abstract

19 Busch ORC, Hop WCJ, Hoynck MAW, et al. Blood transfusions and prognosis in colorectal cancer. *N Engl J Med* 1993;328:1372-1376.

20 Houbiers JGA, Brand A, van de Watering LMG, et al. Randomized controlled trial comparing transfusion of leucocyte-depleted or buffy-coat-depleted blood in surgery for colorectal cancer. *Lancet* 1994;344:573-578.

21 Heiss MM, Mempel W, Jauch KW, et al: Beneficial effect of autologous blood transfusion on infectious complications after colorectal cancer surgery. *Lancet* 1993;342:1328-1333.

22 Jensen LS, Anderson AJ, Christiansen PM, et al: Postoperative infection and natural killer cell function following blood transfusion in patients undergoing elective colorectal surgery. *Br J Surg* 1992;79:513-516.

23 Whyte BM, Swanson CE, Cooper Da. Survival in patients with acquired immunodeficiency syndrome in Australia. *Med J Aust* 1989;150:358-362.

24 Ward JW, Bush TJ, Perkins HJ, et al. The natural history of transfusion-associated infection with human immunodeficiency virus: factors influencing the rate of progression to disease. *N Engl J Med* 1989;321:947-952.

25 Vamvakas, E, Kaplan HS. Early transfusion and length of survival in acquired immune deficiency syndrome: experience with a population receiving medical care at a public hospital. *Transfusion* 1993;33:111-118.

26 Sloand E, Kumar P, Klein HG, et al. Transfusion of blood components to persons infected with HIV-1: relationship to opportunistic infecton. *Transfusion* 1994;34:48-53.

27 Speir E, Modali R, Huan ES, et al. Potential role of human cytomegalovirus and p53 interaction in coronary restenosis. *Science* 1994;265:391-394.

Autologous Blood Procurement: Scope and Liabilities

Lawrence T. Goodnough, MD

Introduction

Autologous blood procurement as a standard of care now has important medical and legal consequences.[1-3] While the net cost of this practice ranges from $60 to $200 per patient,[4] the benefits of autologous blood relative to allogeneic blood have diminished substantially as the blood supply has become increasingly safe.[5,6] As a consequence, autologous blood donation has been found to be poorly cost-effective when compared with other medical interventions,[7-9] and this has led to debate concerning its relative merits.[3,10]

Preoperative autologous blood procurement is regarded as a standard of care for certain elective surgeries,[11,12] particularly for orthopedic and radical prostatectomy procedures.[9,13] Yet, for cardiac surgery, only 42 (7.7%) of 540 patients followed up for transfusion outcomes at 18 institutions had autologous blood available, either by pre-admission donation or by acute normovolemic hemodilution.[14] Furthermore, preoperative autologous blood donation (PAD) in this setting has also been demonstrated to be poorly cost-effective.[8] Decision analysis has shown that approximately 101,000 cardiac surgical patients would need to predonate autologous blood safely to save the life of one patient who would otherwise die of complications related to an allogeneic blood transfusion.[8] Thus, autologous blood donation has not become a standard of care in cardiac surgery, and its safety in this setting is controversial.

There is no good evidence that PAD can be accomplished safely and without mortality before cardiac surgery. In a review of 886 donations in a nonhospital setting by donors not meeting the criteria for allogeneic blood donation (mostly because of their cardiac history), 4.3% of donations were accompanied by reactions, of which four (0.4%) were severe (one transient ischemic attack and three angina episodes).[15] In two smaller hospital-based series, one (1%) of 107 cardiac patients and one (1.2%) of 79 cardiac patients had severe reactions requiring hospitalization.[16,17] In a recent study of 24 patients scheduled for cardiac surgery, Holter monitoring during blood donation demonstrated a significant increase in the duration and intensity of myocardial ischemic events after blood donation.[18] Thus, serious morbid events have been documented to occur during PAD in patients at risk. In addition, there is a defined rate of mortality in cardiac patients who await surgery. In a recent series of cases reported from the Netherlands, 25 (2.2%) of 1124 consecutive patients scheduled for cardiac surgery died before operation.[19] A total of 288 of these patients were on a "medium priority" list, with a mean waiting period of 39 days (which approximates the storage interval for donated blood); two (0.7%) of these patients died before surgery. In an intention-to-treat analysis, any mortality due to progression of cardiac disease during the interval required for autologous blood donation must be considered a complication of PAD. The controversy over the role of PAD in cardiac surgery has been recently debated.[20,21]

Despite published guidelines and consensus conference recommendations that preoperative normovolemic hemodilution (ANH) can be a method of autologous blood procurement,[11,12] the efficacy of this technique has been poorly defined. A case-study analysis in patients undergoing radical prostatectomy demonstrated that in the absence of a defined protocol, ANH has limited efficacy.[22] Subsequently, a prospective ANH approach in which 2000 mL (4 units) hemodilution was performed to lower patients' presurgical Hct level to 28%, followed by retransfusion to maintain perioperative Hct > 25%, was analyzed for 30 consecutive patients and compared with a matched cohort of 30 patients who had predeposited 3 autologous blood units.[23] No difference was found in subsequent allogeneic outcomes: 3 (10%) of 30 patients in each cohort received allogeneic blood. Thus, moderate hemodilution may be an equally effective and less costly alternative to PAD as a blood-conservation strategy, particularly when performed with a defined clinical indicator for blood transfusion.

A similar technique known as blood pooling has been described in cardiac surgery. The removal of 2 autologous blood units at the onset of cardiopulmonary prime was shown in a recent report to reduce subsequent allogeneic blood requirements.[24] However, the perceived advantages[25,26] of fresh whole blood procured by this technique are outweighed by uncertainties (l) regarding its implementation in the large number of patients presenting for surgery who are already anemic, and (2) regarding the intraoperative clinical transfusion indicator for the retransfusion of this blood in patients who already undergo substantial hemodilution related to the crystalloid/colloid pump prime. These issues have prompted both pro and con positions in recent years.[27,28]

References

1. Welch GH, Meehan IT, Goodnough LT. Prudent strategies for elective red cell transfusion. *Ann Intern Med* 1992;116:393-403.

2. Zuck TF. Legal liability for transfusion injury in the acquired immune deficiency syndrome era. *Arch Pathol Lab Med* 1990;114:309-315.

3. Goldfinger D, Haimowitz M. Is autologous blood transfusion worth the cost? Pro. *Transfusion* 1994;75-78.

4. Goodnough LT. Blood transfusion and blood conservation: cost and utilization issues. *Am J Med Qual.* 1994;9:172-183

5. Donahue JG, Munos A, Ness PM, et al. The declining risk of post-transfusion hepatitis C virus infection. *N Engl J Med* 1992;327:369-373.

6. Cumming PD, Wallace EL, Schorr JB, Dodd RY. Exposure of patients to human immunodeficiency virus through the transfusion of blood components that test antibody negative. *N Engl J Med* 1989;321:941-946.

7. Birkmeyer JD, Goodnough LT, Aubuchon JP, et al. The cost-effectiveness of preoperative autologous blood donation for total hip and knee replacement. Transfusion 1993;33:544-551.

8. Birkmeyer JD, Aubuchon JP, Littenberg B, O'Connor GT, Nease RF Jr, Nugent WC, Goodnough LT. Cost-effectiveness of preoperative autologous blood donation in coronary artery bypass grafting. *Ann Thorac Surg* 1994;57:161-169.

9. Goodnough LT, Grishaber JE, Birkmeyer JD, Monk TG, Catalona WJ. Efficacy and cost-effectiveness of autologous blood predeposit in patients undergoing radical prostatectomy procedures. *Urology* 1994;44:226-231.

10. Aubuchon JP, Birkmeyer JD. Is autologous blood transfusion worth the cost? Con. *Transfusion* 1994;34:79-83.

11. National Institutes of Health Consensus Conference. Perioperative red cell transfusion. *JAMA* 1988;260:2700-2705.

12. American College of Physicians. Strategies for elective red cell transfusion. *Ann Intern Med* 1992;116:403-406.

13. Goodnough LT, Shaffron D, Marcus RE. The impact of preoperative autologous blood donation on orthopaedic surgical practice. *Vox Sang* l990;59:65-69.

14. Goodnough LT, Johnston MFM, Toy PTCY, and the TMAA Study Group. The variability of transfusion practice in coronary artery bypass graft surgery. *JAMA* 1991;265:86-90.

15. Aubuchon JP, Popovsky MA. The safety of preoperative autologous blood donation in the nonhospital setting. *Transfusion* 1991:31:513-517.

16. Owings DV, Kruskall MS, Thurer RL, Donovan LM. Autologous blood donations prior to elective cardiac surgery. *JAMA* 1989;262:1963-1968.

17. Dzik WH, Fleisher AG, Ciavarella D, et al. Safety and efficacy of autologous blood donation before elective aortic valve operation. *Ann Thorac Surg* 1992;54:1177-1181.

18. Van Dyck MJ, Baele PL, Leclercq BS, et al. Autologous blood donation before myocardial revascularization: a Holter-electrocardiographic analysis. *J Cardiothorac Vasc Anesth* 1994:8:162-167.

19. Suttorp MJ, Kingma JH, Vos J, et al. Determinants for early mortality in patients awaiting coronary artery bypass graft surgery. *Eur Heart J* 1992;13:238-242.

20. Spiess BD. Autologous blood should be available for elective cardiac surgery. Pro. *J CardiothoracVasc Anesth* 1994;8:231-237.

21. Gravlee GP. Autologous blood collection is not useful for elective coronary artery bypass graft surgery. Con. *J Cardiothorac Vasc Anesth* 1994;8:238-241.

22. Goodnough LT, Grishaber IS, Monk TG, Catalona WJ. Acute preoperative hemodilution in patients undergoing radical prostatectomy: a case study analysis of efficacy. *Anesth Analg* 1994;789:932-937.

23. Monk TG, Goodnough LT, Birkmeyer J, Brecher M, Catalona WJ. Acute preoperative hemodilution is a cost-effective alternative to predeposit in patients undergoing radical prostatectomy. *Transfusion* 1995;35:559-565.

24. Petry AF, Jost T, Sievers H. Reduction of homologous blood requirements by blood pooling at the onset of cardiopulmonary bypass. *J Thorac Cardiovasc Surg* l994;107:1210-1214.

25. Mohr R, Martinowitz U, Lavee J, Arnroch D, Ramot B, Goor DA. The hemostatic effect of transfusing fresh whole blood versus platelet concentrates after cardiac operations. *J Thorac Cardiovasc Surg* 1988;96:530-534.

26. Lavee J, Martinowitz U, Mohr R, Goor DA, Golan M, Langsam J, Malik Z, Savion N. The effect of transfusion of fresh whole blood versus platelet concentrates after cardiac operations. *J Thorac Cardiovasc Surg* 1989;97:204-212.

27. Robblee IA. Blood harvested before cardiopulmonary bypass decreases postoperative blood loss. Pro. *J Cardiothorac Anesth* 1990;4:519-522.

28. Starr NJ. Blood should not be harvested immediately before cardiopulmonary bypass and infused after protamine reversal to decrease blood loss following cardiopulmonary bypass. Con. *J Cardiothorac Anesth* 1990;4:522-525.

The Coagulation System – Physiology and Perioperative Manifestations

Bradford S. Schwartz, MD

If one were to design a hemostatic system, one would want to construct it so that if a tear occurs in the endothelial border of a blood vessel, the system would plug the leak but only at the site of the wound. One would not want the process to extend upward into the vessel to block blood flow or along the endothelial cell lining to areas not wounded. One would want a clot to form only where and when it is needed. Then, when healing is complete and normal endothelial cells have become reestablished, a mechanism would be required to remove the plug (ie blood clot). Otherwise, over the course of a few years, many tiny but eventually noticeable blocks would accumulate and disturb the laminar flow. The process of clearing the clot (fibrinolysis) is enzymatically mediated and, again, one would want it to occur only where and when needed, without the enzymes spilling into the blood and inappropriately digesting other proteins.

HEMOSTASIS

Platelet Adhesion

The hemostatic mechanisms of the human body accomplish the objectives of the optimal design described above. The first phase of hemostasis is often identified as the vascular phase. The initial step in this phase is vasoconstriction, with the blood vessel clamping down to limit blood loss. The next step is that of platelet adhesion, which enables the hemostatic system to recognize the location of the tear in the endothelium. When a tear occurs in a vessel's endothelium, collagen and von Willebrand factor that are immobilized in the subendothelial matrix are exposed to platelets in the blood. Platelets contain receptors for collagen and von Willebrand factor that recognize these proteins only when they are immobilized in the subendothelial matrix, not when they are in solution. Consequently, when the vessel endothelium is intact, platelets coming into contact with endothelial cells simply roll or bounce off the way a tennis ball would bounce off a thick pane of glass. But when platelets contact von Willebrand factor and collagen immobilized in the subendothelial matrix they stick, just as a tennis ball would stick to a panel of Velcro, covering the bare subendothelium with a layer of adherent platelets.

Platelet Aggregation

The next step in the hemostatic process is that of platelet aggregation. The platelets adhering to the subendothelium activate a second set of receptors on their surface and release adenosine diphosphate (ADP) and a variety of adhesive proteins (fibrinogen, fibronectin, von Willebrand factor, vitronectin, thrombospondin). The ADP helps to activate other platelets passing by; the adhesive proteins act as molecular glue, binding both to receptors on the adherent platelets and to receptors on the passing platelets, resulting in a multilayer platelet aggregate at the site of the wound.

Fibrin Formation

There are no covalent bonds holding the platelets together at this point, so if left in this state, the platelet plug formed by platelet aggregation would come apart in a few hours, resulting in late bleeding. The process of blood coagulation, with soluble factors in the blood entering into a chain of reactions that lead to the formation of fibrin, prevents this. Fibrin is a gel with great structural integrity; it acts to sew together the platelet plug to create relative permanence.

Specific properties of platelets and the coagulation system cooperate to ensure that fibrin formation occurs only at the localized site where it is required to initiate wound repair. The surface of resting platelets contains acidic phospholipids with their negative charges directed inward. The inward direction of these negative charges of the resting platelet appears to be sufficiently important so that a specific enzyme exists with the sole role of reversing the orientation of the charge whenever it becomes directed outward. It is only when the platelet becomes activated that the negative charges are allowed to remain on the outside surface of the platelet membrane.

Vitamin K-Dependent Factors

Vitamin K-dependent coagulation factors now come into play, with vitamin K and calcium having essential roles. The coagulation factors possess groups of negatively charged glutamic acids at their N-terminal regions. Vitamin K acts as a cofactor for an enzyme that adds carboxylic acid to the glutamic acid, forming γ-carboxy glutamic acid, with resultant higher-density negative charges. Most of the vitamin K-dependent factors will now have between 9 to 12 of these γ-carboxy glutamic acid groups available for reaction at their N-terminals. Positively charged calcium plays its critical role in blood clotting by binding to the coagulation factors with their negatively charged carboxy glutamic acid groups and inducing a conformational change in the protein such that it can now bind to the surface of the activated platelet. One can think of this as an airplane landing on the deck of an aircraft carrier. The calcium serves to cause the vitamin K-dependent protein to drop its "tailhook," which can then catch the "arrest wire" on the activated platelet surface. Hence, the coagulation proteins stop at the site of the wound, and not elsewhere.

The Coagulation Cascade

The coagulation cascade comes into play next. The best characterized reaction in this cascade involves the activation of prothrombin to thrombin by activated factor X and can be taken as the prototype for all other cascade reactions. The enzyme factor Xa is one of the vitamin K-dependent proteins that binds calcium and becomes bound to a platelet surface. The Xa may now very well be located next to a molecule of prothrombin that is vitamin K-dependent and, therefore, also held on the platelet surface in a dependent manner by calcium and in a position to productively interact with it, activating the prothrombin to form thrombin. This activation of prothrombin by factor Xa is 22 times more likely to occur with both factor Xa and prothrombin held in place on a platelet surface than if the enzyme and substrate were just floating in solution (Fig 1).

Basic Reaction: II $\xrightarrow{\text{Xa}}$ IIa

Enzyme, etc	Relative Reaction Rate
Xa	1.0
Xa, PL	1.0
Xa, Ca^{++}	2.3
Xa, Ca,$^{++}$ PL	22.0

Fig 1. Increase in relative reaction rates of prothrombin to thrombin conversion resulting from complex of the substrate and enzyme with calcium and binding to the phospholipid membrane of the platelet.

Nevertheless, the enzymatic activity of factor Xa on prothrombin with the two molecules to a platelet surface is not as efficient as it would need to be. Each factor Xa or prothrombin can spin in any direction, move around, or align with another complex inappropriately to achieve interaction. Factor Va now enters the picture, acting to further amplify the enzymatic efficiency of this process at the wound site. Factor Va is a nonvitamin K-dependent factor that has its own binding site on the platelet's surface. Factor Va can be thought of as reaching up and grabbing both factor Xa and prothrombin, holding them in place and aligning them correctly so that they have no choice but to have productive interaction (Fig 2). The effect of this interaction involving all components of this particular system has been quantified, showing that it remarkably increases the rate of activation of prothrombin to thrombin by a factor of 278,000 (Fig 3).[1]

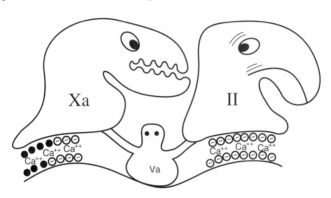

Fig 2. Action of factor Va as a cofactor to stabilize and complex with factor Xa and the substrate factor II on the platelet membrane to further increase the reaction rate of thrombin generation.

Basic Reaction:	II $\longrightarrow$ IIa
	Xa

Enzyme, etc	Relative Reaction Rate
Xa	1.0
Xa, PL	1.0
Xa, Ca^{++}	2.3
Xa, Ca,$^{++}$ PL	22.0
Xa, Ca,$^{++}$ Va	356.0
Xa, Ca,$^{++}$ PL, Va	278,000.0

Fig 3. Action of all the components involved in thrombin generation to increase the relative reaction rate.

This maximal amplification of the reaction rate requires the presence of all the necessary components and their appropriate functioning. Suboptimal vitamin K-dependent carboxylation of the required vitamin K-dependent proteins reduces the efficiency of the reaction. Similarly, the action of the cofactor factor Va is essential; since this cofactor has a half-life of only about 5 hours, it may not be sufficiently available in a patient with impaired liver function, causing the entire system to work suboptimally.

We have learned that once nature hits upon a mechanism that works, it will use it over and over again. Factor Xa is produced when factor X is activated by factor IXa. This reaction is facilitated by a mechanism similar to that involved in the activation of prothrombin. In this case, the nonvitamin K-dependent cofactor VIIIa reaches up from its binding site on a platelet surface and grabs both factor IXa and factor X, aligning them correctly for maximum interaction and generating factor Xa with what is probably also about a 280,000-fold augmentation.

To give real-time examples of how effective this physiologic amplification of coagulation is, a fluid phase two-step coagulation process involving the activation of factor X to Xa followed by the activation of factor II to IIa that would require 3 months would take only 1 second in the unrestricted intact system (Fig 4). That is a major reason blood clots only where it is supposed to—when things work properly.

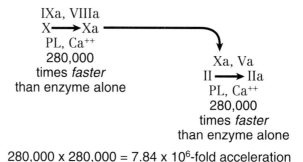

$$280,000 \times 280,000 = 7.84 \times 10^6\text{-fold acceleration}$$

Therefore, what takes *1 second* in the unrestricted intact system requires *3 months* (90.7 days) in a system of enzyme and substrate alone (*ie*, if blood clotted in plasma, not in the activated platelet surface).

Fig 4. Effects of cofactor-dependent complexes on the speed of clot formation.

Another important step in the hemostatic process involves the clotting of fibrinogen to fibrin by thrombin. The result is the formation of a fibrin surface to which the thrombin stays bound. Factor XIII also binds to the fibrin surface; its role in the hemostatic process is to sew the fibrin together so that it does not come apart. Thrombin interacts with factor XIII, with the fibrin surface holding both to facilitate the interaction and to ensure that it occurs only where it is supposed to. Factor XIIIa is then positioned exactly where it is needed, on the fibrin clot, with the result being efficient factor XIIIa-mediated crosslinking of the fibrin molecules.

The essential interactive roles played in hemostasis by both platelets and coagulation factors, as illustrated in the examples discussed above, explain why bleeding will occur in a patient with thrombocytopenia and a normal coagulation system or in a patient with normal platelets but with liver failure.

Fibrinolysis

Once healing has occurred, the fibrin clot must be digested. Two caveats apply: fibrinolysis must occur only when and where it is required; and it must not occur too early.

Both plasminogen, the zymogen precursor to plasmin, and tissue plasminogen activator (t-PA), the enzyme that acts to transform plasminogen to plasmin, are present in flowing blood. Although the t-PA in blood is an active enzyme, when blood is flowing the likelihood of t-PA encountering plasminogen in just the right conformational alignment to permit their interaction is so improbable that virtually no plasminogen is converted to plasmin in the plasma. It is the fibrin surface itself that signals the system to activate fibrinolysis. When a fibrin surface forms, the amino acid lysine protrudes from the fibrin. Plasminogen contains a distinct lysine-binding site, which allows it to bind to lysine on the fibrin surface. Tissue plasminogen activator also has a fibrin-binding site, although its nature is still undefined. When both plasminogen and t-PA bind to the fibrin surface and are appropriately aligned, their interaction occurs readily and plasmin is generated.

Occasionally, the generation of plasmin is somewhat too vigorous. Antifibrinolytic agents such as ε-aminocaproic acid and tranexamic acid are designed to modulate excessive plasmin formation by mimicking lysine, fitting into plasminogen's lysine-binding site and thus preventing the binding of plasminogen to fibrin.

The plasmin generated on a fibrin surface under physiologic conditions is a highly active, broad-spectrum proteolytic enzyme. One can regard it as having roughly the activity of trypsin, definitely not something that should be coursing through a person's veins. Plasmin commonly escapes from its fibrin-binding site because its binding affinity is not very strong. Consequently, there has to be a mechanism to neutralize plasmin when it dissociates from a fibrin clot. A good rule of biochemistry is that for every enzyme there exists a cognate inhibitor. The cognate inhibitor for plasmin is α_2-plasmin inhibitor (also known as α_2-antiplasmin). The plasmin on a fibrin clot is protected against inhibition by α_2-plasmin inhibitor; at this site, the inhibition process takes more than 5 minutes. But when plasmin escapes into solution, α_2-plasma inhibitor exerts its inhibition in 1/100 of a second, which is one of the fastest enzyme/inhibitor interactions in mammalian biology. The system thus protects plasmin when it is working where needed but immediately neutralizes the enzyme when it escapes into solution where it might wreak havoc.

In badly dysregulated states, it is possible to have an excess of plasmin with no α_2-plasmin inhibitor to protect it. This occurs because the molar concentration of plasminogen in the blood is about 2 micromolar, with the potential of making 2 micromoles of plasmin per liter of blood, but the concentration of α_2-plasmin inhibitor is only 1 micromolar. Therefore, antifibrinolytic therapy can be very important in certain circumstances.

The interactions described above that generate an enzyme where needed, restrict the action of the enzyme to that site, and inhibit its effects when the enzyme escapes constitute a model replicated elsewhere in the coagulation system, again reflecting the persistence of successful patterns in biology (Table 1). Thus, antithrombin III does not inhibit thrombin when it is on a clot surface, even in the presence of heparin, but does inhibit thrombin if it escapes into solution. As noted above, nonvitamin K-dependent cofactors act to hold an enzyme and substrate together to facilitate their interaction. If these cofactors were allowed to function on clot surfaces indefinitely, clotting would continue indefinitely. The activated protein C system provides a mechanism that inactivates cofactor Va. However, activated protein C does not inactivate factor Va when the factor is involved in holding enzyme and substrate together but only when it is unencumbered. And plasminogen activator inhibitors do not inhibit plasminogen activators when they are functioning where they are supposed to.

Table 1. Protection From Inactivation: A Repetitive Theme Allowing Properly Placed Reactions to Continue

1. AT-III Inhibition of coagulation enzymes
2. Activated protein C inactivation of factor Va
3. α_2-PI inhibition of plasmin
4. PAI Inhibition of plasminogen activators

AT-III, Antithrombin III; α_2-PI, α_2-plasmin inhibitor; PAI, plasminogen activator inhibitor.

Reference

1. Mann KG, Jenny RJ, Krishnaswamy S. Cofactor proteins in the assembly and expression of blood clotting enzyme complexes. *Annu Rev Biochem* 1988;57:915-956.

Control of Perioperative Bleeding: Blood-Component Therapy

J. Lance Lichtor, MD

This presentation focuses largely on the issues involved in the anesthesiologist's choice of packed cells, platelets, or fresh-frozen-plasma (FFP) when confronted with a patient who is bleeding. Autologous transfusion is always preferred, since it virtually eliminates infectious risks, avoids immunosuppressive effects with regard to tumors or infection, avoids febrile and hemolytic reactions if properly administered, and conserves resources. Preoperative donation, blood salvage, and hemodilution are the three approaches to autologous transfusion in the operating room that will be discussed.

PREOPERATIVE DONATION

It is estimated that approximately 50% of all blood needs could be met by predonation.[1,2] Predonor criteria are less strict than for other donors. Although it is generally agreed that an autologous donor's preoperative hematocrit should be at least 33%, this is still less restrictive than the usual requirement for other donors. Autologous predonation is generally avoided if the patient has neurologic or cardiovascular disease (CD); in series in which autologous donation was attempted in patients with serious CD, it was found to be associated with some incidence of hypotension.[3-5] We see patients preoperatively in our preanesthesia clinic and encourage them to predonate blood if this is deemed appropriate. The donation is done once a week, with the last donation done at least 72 hours prior to surgery. Iron is given to all patients to replenish the iron they lose with their blood donations. Since requirements for predonors are less strict than for other donors, with less complete inquiry into their history and risk behavior, there generally is no crossover; predonated blood does not go into the general pool if it is not used for the patient's operation.

Transfusion with preoperatively donated blood is not risk-free. The most common side effect associated with transfusion is overload, and this probably cannot be avoided. There can be clerical error, whereby the patient accidentally receives allogeneic blood. Also, sepsis may result if the blood is left out too long, and there is the possibility of a hypersensitivity reaction.

INTRAOPERATIVE BLOOD SALVAGE

Intraoperative blood salvage is not appropriate for every surgery.[6] It is inappropriate if the patient has an infection, as we do not want the infectious agent to get into the collected blood. The appropriateness of using blood that shows urine in the field is controversial; we use the blood for salvage if there is only urine and not other signs of transfusion reaction. Blood salvage should also be discontinued when microfibrillar collagen hemostat is used. Since tumor cells may be reinfused, intraoperative salvage is inappropriate for a patient who has a localized tumor; however, when tumor cells are believed to be present throughout the body, using blood salvage probably does not significantly increase the patient's risk.

In intraoperative salvage, the blood is washed and only red cells remain. The hematocrit of this blood is between 50% and 60%, similar to that of blood obtained from the blood bank.

PREOPERATIVE HEMODILUTION

Preoperative hemodilution is less popular as a method of achieving autologous transfusion than preoperative donation and intraoperative blood salvage, largely because it consumes some operating room time and can require extra personnel. With this technique, patients generally are bled down to a hematocrit of 25%. Preoperative hemodilution should be avoided if the patient's hematocrit is less than 33% preoperatively, since less blood can be obtained from the patient in such a circumstance.

The advantages of preoperative hemodilution are (1) normal platelet function is retained since the patient receives back whole blood and not packed cells; (2) hypothermia is avoided if the blood is not refrigerated; and (3) there is less red blood cell loss with operative bleeding because the patient's blood now is more dilute. For an overview of this topic, the reader is referred to several review articles.[7-10]

DESIGNATED DONATIONS

Designated donations offer another approach to obtaining a preoperative supply of blood, although not autologous blood. This approach has fallen out of favor lately because of the clerical burden it imposes, recognition that potential donors among relatives and friends may feel put upon to donate, and the absence of confidentiality and legal protection for donors. Most important, the original rationale for the promotion of designated donations was the belief that the risk of infection would be reduced. But published studies[11] have shown that there is no significant reduction in infectious risk when designated donations are used compared with general blood obtained from the blood bank. Furthermore, the risk of graft-versus-host disease (GVHD) still exists when blood donors are first-degree relatives.

PROTOCOLS FOR BLOOD TRANSFUSION

Blood transfusion is not initiated simply because a patient is bleeding. Our practice is to initially give 3 cc of balanced salt solution for each 1 cc of blood loss. Then when giving packed cells, we give 1 cc for every 2 cc of blood loss.

A decrease in the patient's hematocrit to 20% to 25% often is considered an indication for blood transfusion, but the balance between the patient's oxygen-carrying capacity and oxygen-consumption needs must also be taken into account. A recent study reported on a series of anesthetized patients who were not transfused until their hemoglobin had fallen to about 3 [g/dL] so that their hematocrits then were about 10%.[12] This practice was based on the recognition that the body's oxygen requirement is much lower in anesthetized patients than in awake patients. Young, healthy normocritic patients may be able to tolerate a much lower hematocrit when under anesthesia.

Patients who are chronically anemic (< 7 g/dL hemoglobin) also can tolerate a lower hematocrit. There is no need to transfuse a patient with a hematocrit of 21% if that patient was previously functioning adequately with such a hematocrit.

The amount of packed red blood cells (PRBCs) to be transfused can be calculated by the following formula: hematocrit desired minus hematocrit observed x volume of distribution divided by hematocrit of transfused blood (usually 0.6 or 60%) equals the amount of PRBCs to be transfused (Fig 1).

Figure 1

$$V = V_D \frac{H_d - H_o}{H^+}$$

V_D, Volume of distribution; H_d, Hct desired; H_o, hematocrit observed; H^+, hematocrit of transfused blood.

MAXIMAL SURGICAL BLOOD ORDER SCHEDULE

How much blood should the blood bank hold for patients? The objective is to avoid as much as feasible the holding of unnecessary blood for 24 to 48 hours, with the blood aging and unavailable for other patients during this time. Consequently, a maximal blood order schedule should be developed. Blood-bank personnel, anesthesiologists, and surgeons jointly decide how much blood to hold for different procedures, based on their experience with blood use. Ideally, a crossmatch-to-transfusion ratio will be between 2.1 and 2.7.

Type-and-Screen Indications

For procedures in which blood usually is not required but should neverthe-less be available in the event it is, only a type-and-screen is done. This is similar to a type-and-crossmatch except that it is done with blood that has representative antigens from the larger blood pool available. If a particular antibody is identified in the patient's blood, appropriate units lacking that antigen either are set aside for that patient or, at the least, are determined to be available in the blood bank.

A type-and-screen done when an emergency transfusion is required is 99% effective in preventing a transfusion reaction. Although antigens may occasionally be present in the transfused blood, they usually do not cause severe hemolytic transfusion reactions. If a patient has received a unit of blood after a type-and-screen and then undergoes another procedure for which a type-and-screen is necessary, the type-and-screen must be repeated, as the initial transfusion may have introduced antigens to which new antibodies have developed.

Type-and-Complete Crossmatch Indication

A type and complete crossmatch ideally is done for all nonemergent transfusion. One reason for this is that there may be donor cell antigens that are not present on screening cells. Additionally, the type-and-crossmatch involves a form of duplication that protects against both human error and the possibility of a reaction failure that may occur with a type-and-screen.

Partial-Crossmatch Indication

For an emergency transfusion, the most desirable procedure is to do a partial crossmatch, which includes an ABO-Rh type and immediate phase crossmatch between the patient serum and donor RBCs. This takes about 1 to 5 minutes and eliminates the risk of serious hemolytic reactions.

Type-Specific, Non-Crossmatched Blood

Next in preference would be to use type-specific but non-crossmatched blood. Of course, it is essential to be sure of the patient's blood type; the rec-ollections of relatives or friends about past records cannot be trusted. If the patient's type is accurately established, there is only a 1 in 1,000 incidence of an unexpected antibody being present. Data from the Vietnam War experience indicate that type-specific blood was administered with minimal reactions, and no hemolytic transfusion reaction. The least desirable procedure in the emergent situation is to use type O Rh negative blood that is non-crossmatched. Some O donors have gamma G immunoglobulin (IgG), gamma M immunoglobulin (IgM), or anti-A or anti-B, or AB, so that a type of graft-versus-host reaction occurs. This reaction is less likely with packed cells than with whole blood, since there is less plasma present to contain the IgG or IgM.

BASICS OF BLOOD ADMINISTRATION
Solutions and Filters Recommendations
Packed cells are rather viscous, raising the problem of what solution to add. Hypoosmolar fluids (eg, D5-water) are to be avoided because they cause lysis of cells. Calcium-containing fluids (eg, lactated Ringer's solution) may cause clotting and should be avoided. Saline solution, or isomolar noncalcium electrolyte solution, should be used instead. For filtration, we generally use 170-micron filters, changing the filter after every 4 units of blood stored for more than l0 days or after 8 units of blood stored for less than l0 days. The practice by some of using a smaller filter of 25 or 40 microns, such as the Pall Ultipor 40um filter, to prevent febrile reactions is not cost-effective in the absence of a previous febrile reaction to transfusion.

In contrast to administering blood on the wards, blood given in the operating room has to be warmed. Administering unwarmed blood directly to the heart through a central line can cause hypothermia and cardiac arrest.

Metabolic Changes Involving Calcium
Possible metabolic changes in anesthetized patients should be considered. A normal liver can metabolize calcium citrate rather quickly, so the practice by some of giving calcium prophylactically to avoid hypotension whenever blood is administered at a rate faster than 1 unit every 5 minutes is controversial. Certainly, if the liver is not functioning properly, as often occurs in liver transplant surgery, the patient is unable to metabolize calcium, becomes hypotensive, and requires calcium. But this probably is not true when liver function is normal. Issues of potassium load, acid-base balance, and hypothermia are no different in the operating room than elsewhere.

Dilutional Thrombocytopenia Indications
The more blood transfused, and particularly the more units of PRBCs, the more likely the occurrence of dilutional thrombocytopenia. This possibility must be considered in the presence of clinical coagulopathy. A diagnosis of dilutional thrombocytopenia is difficult to make in the operating room because there is no really rapid means of measuring platelets. Consequently, if much blood has been transfused and the patient is oozing, we administer some platelets. A patient with altered platelet function because of drugs, cardiopulmonary bypass, or uremia may tend to bleed more. Therefore, platelet administration is recommended when bleeding occurs in the presence of thrombocytopenia or abnormal platelet function.

One platelet concentrate increases the patient's platelet count by 5,000 to 10,000. No filter smaller than 170 microns should be used because it will remove platelets. Similarly, small needles or angiocatheters will not permit the passage of platelets; platelets should be administered through the largest line that is available.

Dilution of Factors V and VIII
Transfusion can also lead to dilution of factors V and VIII. In whole blood, factor V is decreased to 15% of normal and factor VIII to 50% of normal af-

ter 2l days of storage, and PRBCs contain even less of these factors. Five percent to 20% of normal levels of factor V and 30% of normal levels of factor VIII are required for hemostasis. Fortunately, a monitor (Ciba Corning) is available that can be used in the operating room to measure prothrombin time (PT) and partial thromboplastin time (PTT) and requires only about 2 minutes to obtain a reading. When there is generalized bleeding and the PTT is >l.5 with the platelet count normal (>70,000), the administration of FFP is indicated. Even with patients who have generalized bleeding but whose PTT is not quite over 1.5, administering FFP may reduce bleeding.

OTHER TRANSFUSION-RELATED REACTIONS
Other factors to consider when transfusing blood are hypotension and hypoperfusion, disseminated intravascular coagulation (DIC), and hemolytic toxic reactions. A febrile reaction is the most common problem associated with transfusion, usually secondary to leukocytes. Allergic or infectious reactions attributable to the transfusion of plasma can occur, as can a hemolytic reaction to transfused erythrocytes.

Increased temperature should be avoided in anesthetized patients. This is not generally a problem in the operating room, particularly since patients are cold to begin with. But to prevent increased temperature, particularly in patients who have had previous febrile reactions, leukocyte-poor RBCs and prophylactic antipyretics can be given and microaggregate filters used. Major signs and symptoms of a hemolytic transfusion reaction indicating that the administration of blood should be discontinued include flushing, hypotension, abnormal bleeding, urticaria, and hemoglobinuria. Others are back pain, nausea, pruritus, chills, and fever. Although these signs and symptoms may be readily apparent outside the operating room, many may be missed in anesthetized patients. Back pain or nausea cannot be determined in an anesthetized patient, and pruritus, chills, and fever are not usually evident. Consequently, given the choice, rather than just administering a unit or two of blood in the operating room before the patient goes to recovery, it is preferable to administer any needed blood when the patient is in the recovery room and awake, assuming that the hematocrit is accurate.

References

1.   Nicholls MD, Janu MR, Davies VJ, Wedderburn CE. Autologous blood transfusion for elective surgery. *Med J Aust* 1986;144:396-399.

2.   Mercuriali F, Inghilleri G, Biffi E, et al. The potential role of oxygen-carrying products in autologous blood transfusion protocols. *Artif Cells, Blood Sub Immobil Biotechnol* 1994;22:245-251. Review.

3.   Van Dyck MJ, Baele PL, Leclercq P, Bertrand M, Brohet C. Autologous blood donation before myocardial revascularizaion: a Holter-electrocardiographic analysis. *J Cardiothorac Vasc Anesth* 1994;8:162-167.

4.   Goldfinger D, Capon S, Czer L, et al. Safety and efficacy of preoperative donation of blood for autologous use by patients with end-stage heart and lung disease who are awaiting organ transplantation. *Transfusion* 1993;33:336-340.

5.   Spiess BD, Sassetti R, McCarthy RJ, Narbone RF, Tuman KJ, Ivankovich AD. Autologous blood donation: hemodynamics in a high-risk patient population. *Transfusion* 1992;32:17-22.

6.   Dzik WH, Sherburne B. Intraoperative blood salvage: medical controversies. *Transf Med Rev* 1990;4:208-235. Review.

7.   Tawes RL Jr. Alternatives to homologous blood transfusion. *Semin Vasc Surg* 1994;7:72-75. Review.

8.   Intaglietta M. Hemodilution and blood substitutes. *Artif Cells Blood Sub Immobil Biotechnol* 1994;22:137-144. Review.

9.   Spahn DR, Leone BJ, Reves JG, Pasch T. Cardiovascular and coronary physiology of acute isovolemic hemodilution: a review of nonoxygen-carrying and oxygen-carrying solutions. *Anesth Analg* 1994;78:1000-1021. Review.

10. Stehling L, Zauder HL. Controversies in transfusion medicine. Perioperative hemodilution: pro. *Transfusion* 1994;34:265-268. Review.

11. Cordell RR, Yalon VA, Cigahn-Haskell C, McDonough BP, Perkins HA. Experience with 11,916 designated donors. *Transfusion* 1986;26:484-486.

12. Fontana JL, Welborn L, Mongan PD, Sturm P, Martin G, Bunger R. Oxygen consumption and cardiovascular function in children during profound intraoperatve normovolemic hemodilution. *Anesth Analg* 1995;80:219-225.

Control of Perioperative Bleeding: The Surgical Perspective

Michael Sobel, MD

Ensuring adequate hemostasis is a routine part of the surgeon's everyday tasks. The relatively rare instances of uncontrolled hemorrhaging encountered are both challenging and extremely frustrating. Meeting this challenge requires a thorough understanding of the coagulation cascade.

CRITICAL ISSUES IN THE COAGULATION CASCADE

Figure l depicts the plasma protein coagulation cascade in a slightly modified form to emphasize critical issues. The body's clotting mechanisms essentially are directed toward generating high local concentrations of thrombin. This is achieved through the assembly of two complexes. The prothrombinase complex includes platelet phospholipids, activated factor X, factor Va, and calcium; this complex converts prothrombin to thrombin. Functioning of the prothrombinase complex is preceded by that of the factor X activating complex, composed of a very analogous collection of factors and cofactors.

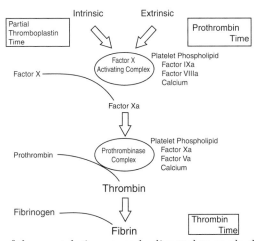

Fig 1. Components of the coagulation cascade directed towards thrombin generation and formation of fibrin clot. Specific in vitro laboratory tests can identify abnormalities at different parts of the cascade, and these are outlined in the figure. (Reproduced with permission from Sobel, M. Callow and Ernst, eds. *Vascular Surgery: Theory and Practice.* Appleton Lange, © 1995.)

Platelets are also central to normal hemostasis; they are the first blood component to arrive at sites of vascular injury, where they release procoagulant proteins and vasoconstrictors. With disruption of the vascular endothelium, subendothelial elements that include collagen and von Willebrand factor are exposed. Platelets adhere to these sites and undergo both metabolic and structural changes, changing from their resting discoid shape into activated plump cells with pseudopodia extending from their surfaces. These changes serve to recruit additional platelets to a growing thrombus.

The platelet membrane also undergoes changes and serves as the scaffold for the assembly of the factor X activating and prothrombinase complexes. These complexes of activated clotting factors assemble on the platelet membrane surface, thus achieving greater enzymatic efficiency than possible with their components in solution. The nonvitamin-K-dependent factors V and VIII contribute to complex formation by helping to align complex components as they settle onto the platelet membrane.

HEMOSTATIC INTERVENTIONS

Tools available to the surgeon to promote hemostasis include cautery techniques, tissue adhesives, and physicochemical and physiologic agents.

Cautery

Cautery is one of the oldest and still most effective of hemostatic tools. It desiccates tissue and destroys and alters proteins, and in so doing welds and seals damaged vessels.

Modern electrocautery originated in the 1920s with William T. Bovie, an engineer and physicist. Bovie was the first to appreciate the significance of earlier turn-of-the-century observations that very high-frequency oscillating currents could pass through the human body without significant pain or injury and could generate local heat in the tissues. With the encouragement and practical help of Harvey Cushing, Bovie developed a machine in the 1930s that was the precursor to our modern electrocoagulation equipment.

The main effect of both standard electrocautery and laser cautery is to achieve localized and controlled delivery of heat to denature proteins and seal vessels. The argon beam electrocoagulator also provides a stream of argon gas that clears the operative field of blood, which often impedes the efficacy of the coagulating current. The argon beam electrocoagulator also replaces oxygen in the atmosphere of the local coagulation site, allowing for a more homogenous, uniform delivery of current and a more superficial injury. The principal issues with all cautery techniques involve the relative balance between hemostatic efficacy and degree of extended tissue damage and include matters of cost and convenience as related to a specific application, be it neurosurgery, liver transplantation, or vascular surgery.

Tissue Adhesives

Fibrin glue probably is the most important and popular of available tissue adhesives. Fibrin glue is assembled instantly by the mixing of essential ingredients at the site of bleeding in the surgical wound. These include a source of human fibrinogen, bovine thrombin, and calcium. Human fibrinogen can be supplied by cryoprecipitate or fresh-frozen plasma. (In Europe, several forms of pasteurized human fibrinogen are available.) Fibrin glue provides all the exogenous substrates necessary for clot formation and thus results in an "instant" mature fibrin thrombus. Useful supplements to fibrin glue include microcrystalline collagen and aprotinin, which can prevent early lysis of the formed clot. Fibrin glue has been used effectively to achieve hemostasis in localized bleeding in hemophiliacs, at sites of vascular suture lines in hemostatically compromised patients, and in surgery of the liver and spleen.

Physicochemical Agents

Physicochemical agents commonly used to promote hemostasis include gelatin foam and oxidized cellulose. Gelatin foam has no intrinsic procoagulant effect; rather, it functions as a sponge, serving to accumulate and retain activated coagulation factors at the site of bleeding. Its effectiveness is further increased when it is saturated with bovine thrombin.

Oxidized cellulose initiates coagulation by the contact activation pathway and provides a meshwork for platelet adherence and the stabilization of fibrin polymers. Oxidized cellulose works because it is highly acidic; consequently, it is not optimally combined with thrombin, which, as a natural enzyme, requires a neutral pH for greatest efficacy. Oxidized cellulose also has antibacterial properties.

Physiologic Agents
Topical thrombin and bovine collagen are highly useful hemostatic agents. Applied directly to a bleeding site, thrombin bypasses all but the final phase of coagulation, that of fibrin formation. Purified bovine thrombin is used most commonly for this purpose. It is useful whenever the earlier phases of the coagulation cascade are inhibited or deficient, as in a heparinized patient, a patient who has been taking warfarin, or a patient with vitamin K deficiency. Rarely, repeated massive exposure to topical thrombin can induce antibodies to thrombin and factor V, resulting in pseudohemophilia or acquired hemophilia.

My experience suggests that applying topical thrombin also can be used as an informal in vivo diagnostic test to suggest the nature of the problem posed by a bleeding patient. Thus, if the thrombin applied to the operative field does not induce normal clot formation, then fibrinogen may be deficient. The formation of clots of poor quality, loose and friable, may indicate the presence of excessive heparin, defective fibrin polymerization, or thrombocytopenia. The presence of excessive heparin constitutes just a stoichiometric problem, requiring administration of more topical thrombin. Defective fibrin polymerization may occur in patients with liver failure who may have defective fibrinogen molecules that do not polymerize properly. In cases of disseminated intravascular coagulation (DIC) or pathologic fibrinolysis, very elevated levels of fibrin degradation products can interfere with polymerization. Thrombocytopenia can be responsible for poor clot quality, since platelets normally contribute significantly to the final phases of clot retraction and solidification and add to the firmness of the final clot. Finally, the rapid lysing of clots once they are formed suggests the possibility of pathologic fibrinolysis.

Collagen is a natural potent activator and adhesive for platelets. Purified bovine collagen is available as sheets, pads, and powders suitable for application to a variety of bleeding sites. It is especially useful when platelet function or number is diminished, as in cardiopulmonary bypass or massive transfusion. The combined use of collagen and topical thrombin is synergistic, activating both platelets and the coagulation cascade.

ANALYSIS OF INTRAOPERATIVE BLEEDING
In a simple paradigm for the analysis of intraoperative bleeding, problems may be differentiated as either mechanical/technical or hematologic/ biochemical. Mechanical/technical problems may involve leaky needle holes or raw bleeding surfaces of solid organs. Hematologic/biochemical problems may involve platelet dysfunction or thrombocytopenia in transplantation or coronary bypass, pathologic fibrinolysis in liver failure, or DIC. It is the physician's task to use the hemostatic agent(s) or technique(s) appropriate to the cause of the bleeding.

Control of Perioperative Bleeding: Pharmacologic Agents

Marcus E. Carr Jr, MD, PhD

Recent years have seen a proliferation of agents designed to aid surgical hemostasis without resorting to blood-component transfusion. These drugs have a broad spectrum of activities, but can be grouped into three categories: antifibrinolytics, antithrombins, and topical hemostatic agents (the Table).

Pharmacologic Agents That Aid Hemostasis		
Antifibrinolytics	**Antithrombins**	**Topical Hemostatics**
ε-Aminocaproic acid	Hirudin r-Hirudin Modified hirudin	Fibrin glue (adhesive)
Tranexamic acid	Argatroban (MD-805)	Absorbable collagen (INSTAT)
Aprotinin	Heparin	Calcium alginate (hemostatic swab)
	Low-molecular-weight heparin	Topical thrombin

Antifibrinolytic Agents

Aprotinin, ε-aminocaproic acid (EACA), and tranexamic acid (AMCHA) are the three antifibrinolytic agents that have dominated recent clinical studies. Aprotinin, molecular weight 6512 daltons, is a broad-spectrum serine protease inhibitor that was first isolated from bovine lymph node in 1930.[1] At low concentrations (50 kallikrein inhibitor units [KIU]/mL), aprotinin inhibits trypsin and plasmin. At high concentrations (200 KIU/mL), aprotinin also inhibits tissue and plasma kallikrein.[2] It was first used in cardiopulmonary bypass (CPB) patients in an effort to inhibit plasmin-induced complement activation. With such applications, decreased bleeding and transfusion requirements were noted. These results were subsequently confirmed in multiple studies, and an exhaustive review of aprotinin's therapeutic potential has been published.[3,4]

Aprotinin

Aprotinin is postulated to improve hemostasis during CPB by reducing CPB-induced platelet dysfunction.[5] It is thought to accomplish this by suppressing kallikrein and plasmin activities. During CPB, exposure of plasma to the synthetic surfaces of the CPB circuit activates coagulation contact factors (Fig 1). Activated factor XII promotes the conversion of prothrombin to thrombin through the intrinsic pathway. Once activated, thrombin causes platelet activation and degranulation. Kallikrein, which is also activated during the contact phase of coagulation, promotes conversion of plasminogen to plasmin. When activated, plasmin cleaves glycoprotein 1b (GP1b) receptors from the platelet surface. Platelet degranulation leads to an acquired storage pool defect, while loss of GPlb causes an acquired adhesion defect. Platelet dysfunction results. By inhibiting kallikrein and plasmin, aprotinin decreases both thrombin generation and GPlb cleavage.[6] This scenario may explain platelet preservation noted with aprotinin.

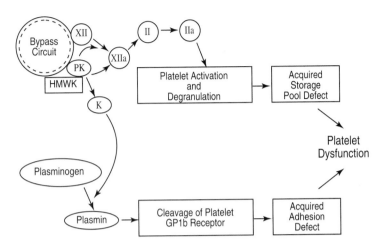

Fig 1. Proposed mechanism for development of platelet dysfunction during cardiopulmonary bypass. Aprotinin may interrupt process by inhibiting kallikrein (K) and plasmin. HMWK, High-molecular-weight kininogen; XII, factor XII (Hageman factor), II; factor II (thrombin).

Other functions attributed to aprotinin include reducing heparin binding to platelets and inhibition of protein C.[7,8] Inhibition of protein C, a natural anticoagulant, enhances coagulation and reduces fibrinolysis. Additional clinical studies have demonstrated decreased blood transfusion requirements when aprotinin is used during liver transplantation. Although the optimal dose has not been established, repeated hourly boluses of 0.5 million KIU or 0.5 million KIU/h by continuous infusion decrease blood loss and transfusion requirements during CPB and orthotopic liver transplant (OLT).[9]

Although unusual, several side effects of aprotinin have been reported. Allergic, anaphylactic reactions occur in less than 0.1% of cases.[10] Drug interactions are more common. Aprotinin reduces the fibrinolytic response to tissue plasminogen activator (t-PA) or streptokinase.[11] The combination of aprotinin and angiotensin-converting enzyme (ACE) inhibitors can result in increased blood pressure.[12] When used with heparin, aprotinin causes additional prolongation of the activated clotting time (ACT) and the activated partial thromboplastin time (aPTT).[13,14] Other infrequently reported complications include worsening of renal insufficiency, early coronary graft closure, and increased risk of perioperative myocardial infarction.[15]

ε-Aminocaproic Acid; Tranexamic Acid
ε-Aminocaproic acid and AMCHA are lysine analogues that inhibit fibrinolysis. Interestingly, both EACA (131 daltons) and AMCHA (157 daltons) accelerate conversion of plasminogen to plasmin. Inhibition of fibrinolysis occurs at the subsequent substrate binding step where plasmin-fibrin(ogen) complex formation is blocked.[16] Until recently, these agents have been primarily used to reduce mucosal membrane bleeding in hemophilia and von Wille-

brand's disease. ε-Aminocaproic acid also decreases bleeding in thrombocytopenic oncology patients. Upon demonstration that fibrinolysis associated with liver transplantation is usually a primary event (ie, not secondary to disseminated intravascular coagulation), application of EACA was deemed appropriate and has been shown to decrease transfusion requirements.[17] Prophylactic use of EACA in CPB reduces blood loss at 24 hours, decreases transfusion requirements, and does not appear to induce a hyperthrombotic state.[18] When tested, AMCHA appears to be equivalent to EACA. When combined with 1-deamino-(8-D-arginine)-vasopressin (DDAVP), EACA did not decrease intraoperative blood loss but did decrease postoperative bleeding and transfusion requirements.[18] At a dose of 100 mg EACA/kg body weight, EACA reduces bleeding, transfusion requirements and the incidence of intracranial hemorrhage in neonates undergoing extracorporeal membrane oxygenation (ECMO).[19] Recent studies have demonstrated that the previously suggested loading dose of 5 gm followed by 1 gm every hour is excessive and that as little as 250 mg as a single dose is effective for most prophylactic uses. As with aprotinin, the therapeutic effects of EACA and AMCHA in CPB are felt to be due to decreased fibrinolysis and sparing of platelet GPIb.

Antithrombin Agents
Heparin
Heparin, the prototype IV anticoagulant, works by augmenting the antithrombin effects of antithrombin III. Three primary advantages of heparin are that it acts rapidly, it can be rapidly reversed by administering protamine sulfate, and it is relatively inexpensive. Disadvantages of heparin include the need for frequent laboratory monitoring, the potential for life-threatening heparin-associated thrombocytopenia (HAT), and problems associated with the use of protamine as an antidote. These problems have spurred the development of low-molecular-weight heparins (LMWHs) that do not require frequent monitoring, of novel antithrombin compounds that are unrelated to heparin and can be used in patients with HAT, and of alternatives to protamine reversal of heparin. Low-molecular-weight heparins are an interesting and useful class of compounds whose properties have been reviewed elsewhere[20] and will not be addressed here.

Hirudin
New antithrombin agents include proteins isolated from other organisms and synthetic peptides designed to inhibit serine proteases. Hirudin, a protein derived from leeches, has recently been produced in large quantities by recombinant technology.[21] Circulating levels of 2 to 20 μg/mL (0.1-1.0 mg/kg) are antithrombotic in animal models of stasis thrombosis.[22] In a rabbit model, blood loss from ear incisions was not increased at hirudin levels up to 20 μg/mL. At 50 and 100 μg/mL (2.5-5.0 mg/kg), bleeding was increased and was equivalent to that seen with 1.25 to 2.50 mg/kg of heparin. Although the half-life of hirudin is relatively short, there is no rapid antidote for reversal. Hirudin is not neutralized by platelet factor 4 (PF4), protamine sulfate, other polycationic agents, or heparinase.[22] Bleeding in association with hirudin can be corrected using activated prothrombin complex conjugates and may be responsive to recombinant factor VIIa.[22] The former agent does carry some thrombotic risk.

Argatroban

A series of potent synthetic antithrombins are in development. Argatroban (MD-805), an arginine derivative, is a potent antithrombin (Ki - 0.019 µmol) that lacks antifibrinolytic activity.[23] It has been used successfully in the treatment of AT-III-deficient patients and during hemodialysis in heparin-intolerant patients. Perhaps its most promising potential indication is in patients suffering from HAT. In this setting, argatroban produces anticoagulation, inhibits heparin-induced platelet aggregation, and inhibits binding of antiplatelet antibody to platelets. RO46-6240 (Hoffmann-LaRoche) is another recently reported synthetic agent with therapeutic promise.[24] Its anticoagulant properties appear comparable to that of heparin and hirudin.

Developments in Heparin Reversal

Although standard procedure, protamine reversal of heparin has become the subject of intense investigation. Protamine administration causes activation of the complement system and the cyclooxygenase pathway, adverse hemodynamic effects, and occasional pulmonary hemorrhage and edema.[25-28] One approach to avoiding these problems has been to reduce the protamine dose. A single dose of 2 mg/kg has been found to be as effective as the same dose repeated. A new reversal ratio of 0.6 mg protamine per 1 mg heparin appears to be effective.[29] Finally, titration of heparin reversal utilizing monitors such as the HEMOCHRON system results in decreased protamine use. Alternatives to protamine include methylene blue and platelet factor 4 (PF4). Recombinant PF4 (rPF4) has been produced, and heparin reversal with this agent reportedly avoids the decline in platelet count, white cell count and complement seen with protamine use.[30]

Appropriate Clinical Uses of DDAVP

l-Deamino-(8-D-arginine)-vasopressin, a synthetic analogue of antidiuretic hormone, causes release of pre-formed von Willebrand factor (vWF) and FVIII.[31] It has demonstrated utility in the treatment of mild hemophilia and von Willebrand's disease (vWD).[32] Vasopressin also improves hemostasis in patients with uremic platelet dysfunction.[33] The ability to improve qualitative platelet dysfunction prompted trials of DDAVP during CPB.[34] While several early trials were encouraging, subsequent trials have failed to demonstrate a consistent response.[35] Positive responses have been most consistently demonstrated in complex cardiac operations and in patients with aspirin-associated post-CPB hemorrhage.[36] Doses of 10 µg/m^2 or 0.3 µg/kg have decreased blood loss by 40% and transfusion requirements by 34% in selected patients.

Topical Hemostatics

Topical hemostatic agents include topical thrombin,[37,38] absorbable collagen (INSTAT),[39] vasoconstricting agents (oxymetazoline),[40] hemostatic swabs (calcium alginate),[41] and biologic adhesives (fibrin glue).[42] Vasoconstricting agents and collagen hemostatics have been used with success in ear, nose, and throat (ENT) surgery and in oral surgery. Calcium alginate swabs have been reported to decrease blood loss and shorten operative time in patients undergoing cholecystectomy and simple mastectomy.[41] Like its precursor, topical thrombin, fibrin glue has a multitude of applications. While several commercial products are available in Europe, use in the United States has been confined to preparations of autologous fibrin glue. The glue is prepared at the time of application by mixing bovine thrombin, calcium, and concentrated fibrinogen. Numerous studies have documented the efficacy of fibrin glue in cardiovascular, ENT, and neurologic surgical procedures. The material aids hemostasis, promotes tissue sealing, does not cause foreign body reaction, and is completely absorbed. Once the problem of potential viral contamination is handled, fibrin glue is certain to gain increasing acceptance.

Conclusion

Developments of the last 15 years have enabled surgeons, anesthesiologists, and medical consultants to apply an increasingly sophisticated array of agents to treat and arrest perioperative hemorrhage.

References

1. Kraut E, Frey E, Werle E. Über die Inaktivierung des Kallikreins. Hoppe-Seyler's *Zeitschrift für Physiologische Chemie* 1930;192:1-21.

2. Fritz H, Wunderer G. Biochemistry and applications of aprotinin, the kallikrein inhibitor from bovine organs. *Arzneimittel-Forschung* 1983;33(4):479-494 .

3. Hardy JF, Desroches J. Natural and synthetic antifibrinolytics in cardiac surgery. *Can J Anaesth* 1992;39(4):353-365.

4. Royston D. High-dose aprotinin therapy: a review of the first five years' experience. *J Cardiothorac Vasc Anesth* 1992;6:76-100.

5. Harker LA. Bleeding after cardiopulmonary bypass. *N Engl J Med* 1986;314:446-448.

6. van Oeveren W, Harder MP, Roozendaal KJ. Aprotinin protects platelets against the initial effect of cardiopulmonary bypass. *J Thorac Cardiovasc Surg* 1990;99:788-797.

7. John LC, Rees GM, Kovacs IB. Reduction of heparin binding to and inhibition of platelets by aprotinin. *Ann Thorac Surg* 1993;55(5):1175-1179.

8. España F, Estelle SA, Griffin J. Aprotinin (Trasylol) is a competitive inhibitor of activated protein C. *Thromb Res* 1989;56:751-756.

9. Bechstein WO, Riess H, Blumhardt G, et al. Aprotinin in orthotopic liver transplantation. *Semin Thromb Hemost* 1993;19(3):262-267.

10. Taylor KM. Aprotinin therapy in cardiac surgery. *Therapy Express* 1991;37:1-5.

11. Wiman B. On the reaction of plasmin or plasmin-streptokinase complex with aprotinin or alpha 2-antiplasmin. *Thromb Res* 1980;17(1-2):143-152.

12. Overlack A, Stumpe KO, Kuhnert M, et al. Evidence for participation of kinins in the antihypertensive effect of converting enzyme inhibition. *Klin Wochenschr* 1981;59(2):69-74.

13. Royston D, Bidstrup BP, Taylor KM, Sapsford RM. Reduced blood loss following open heart surgery with aprotinin (Trasylol) is associated with an increase in intraoperative activated clotting time (ACT). *J Cardiothorac Anesth* 1989;3(5 suppl 1):80.

14. Dietrich W, Spannagl M, Jochum M. Influence of high-dose aprotinin treatment on blood loss and coagulation patterns in patients undergoing myocardial revascularisation. *Anesthesiology* 1990;73:1119-1126.

15. Cosgrove DM, Heric B, Lytle BW, et al. Aprotinin therapy for reoperative myocardial revascularization: a placebo-controlled study. *Ann Thorac Surg* 1992;54(6):1031-1036.

16. Verstraete M. Clinical application of inhibitors of fibrinolysis. *Drugs* 1985;29(3):236-261.

17. Kang Y. Clinical use of synthetic antifibrinolytic agents during liver transplantation. *Semin Thromb Hemost* 1993;19(3):258-261.

18. Arom KV, Emery RW. Decreased postoperative drainage with addition of epsilon-aminocaproic acid before cardiopulmonary bypass. *Ann Thorac Surg* 1994;57(5): 1108-1112.

19. Wilson JM, Bower LK, Fackler JC, Beals DA, Bergus BO, Kevy SV. Aminocaproic acid decreases the incidence of intracranial hemorrhage and other hemorrhagic complications of ECMO. *J Pediatr Surg* 1993;28(4):536-540.

20. Hirsh J, Levine MN. Low molecular weight heparin. *Blood* 1992; 79(1): 1-17.

21. Fareed J, Walenga JM, Hoppensteadt DA, Pifarré R. Development perspectives for recombinant hirudin as an antithrombotic agent. *Biol Clin Hematol* 1989;11:143-152.

22. Fareed J, Walenga JM, Pifarré R, Hoppensteadt D, Koza M. Some objective considerations for the neutralization of the anticoagulant actions of recombinant hirudin. *Haemostasis* 1991;21(suppl 1):64-72.

23. Matsuo T, Kario K, Kodama K, Okamoto S. Clinical application of the synthetic thrombin inhibitor, argatroban (MD-805). *Semin Thromb Hemost* 1992;18(2):155-160.

24. Gast A, Tschopp TB, Schmid G, Hilpert K, Ackermann J. Inhibition of clot-bound and free (fluid-phase thrombin) by a novel synthetic thrombin inhibitor (RO46-6240), recombinant hirudin and heparin in human plasma. *Blood Coagul Fibrinolysis* 1994;5:879-887.

25. Lowenstein E, Johnston WE, Lappas DG, et al. Catastrophic pulmonary vasoconstriction associated with protamine reversal of heparin. *Anesthesiology* 1983;59(5):470-473.

26. Holland CL, Singh AK, McMaster PR, Fang W. Adverse reactions to protamine sulfate following cardiac surgery. *Clin Cardiol* 1984;7(3):157-162.

27. Morel DR, Zapol WM, Thomas SJ. C5a and thromboxane generation associated with pulmonary vaso- and bronchoconstriction during protamine reversal of heparin. *Anesthesiology* 1987;66:597-604.

28. Weiss ME, Nyhan D, Peng Z, et al. Association of protamine IgE and IgG antibodies with life-threatening reactions to intravenous protamine. *N Engl J Med* 1989;320:886-892.

29. Wright SJ, Murray WB, Hampton WA, Hargovan H. Calculating the protamine-heparin reversal ratio: a pilot study investigating a new method. *J Cardiothorac Vasc Anesth* 1993;7(4):416-421.

30. Cook JJ, Niewiarowski S, Yan Z, et al. Platelet factor 4 efficiently reverses heparin anticoagulation in the rat without adverse effects of heparin-protamine complexes. *Circulation* 1992;85(3):1102-1109.

31. Mannucci PM, Pareti FI, Ruggeri ZM. Enhanced factor VIII activity in von Willebrand's disease. *N Engl J Med* 1974;290(22):1259. Letter.

32. Mannucci PM, Ruggeri ZM, Pareti FI, Capitanio A. 1-Deamino-8-D-arginine vasopressin: a new pharmacological approach to the management of haemophilia and von Willebrand's disease. *Lancet* 1977;1(8017):869-872.

33. Mannucci PM, Remuzzi G, Pusineri F, et al. Deamino-8-D-arginine vasopressin shortens the bleeding time in uremia. *N Engl J Med* 1983;308(1):8-12.

34. Salzman EW, Weinstein MJ, Reilly D, Ware JA. Adventures in hemostasis: desmopressin in cardiac surgery. *Arch Surg* 1993;128(2):212-217.

35. Temeck BK, Bachenheimer LC, Katz NM, Coughlin SS, Wallace RB. Desmopressin acetate in cardiac surgery: a double-blind, randomized study. *South Med J* 1994;87(6):611-615.

36. Chard RB, Kam CA, Nunn GR, Johnson DC, Meldrum Hanna W. Use of desmopressin in the management of aspirin-related and intractable haemorrhage after cardiopulmonary bypass. *Aust N Z J Surg* 1990;60(2):125-128.

37. Ofodile FA, Sadana MK. The role of topical thrombin in skin grafting. *J Natl Med Assoc* 1991;83(5):416-418.

38. Ortel TL, Charles LA, Keller FG, et al. Topical thrombin and acquired coagulation factor inhibitors: clinical spectrum and laboratory diagnosis. *Am J Hematol* 1994;45(2):128-135.

39. Green JG, Durham TM. Application of INSTAT hemostat in the control of gingival hemorrhage in the patient with thrombocytopenia: a case report. *Oral Surg Oral Med Oral Pathol* 1991;71(1):27-30.

40. Riegle EV, Gunter JB, Lusk RP, Muntz HR, Weiss KL. Comparison of vasoconstrictors for functional endoscopic sinus surgery in children. *Laryngoscope* 1992;102(7):820-823.

41. Blair SD, Jarvis P, Salmon M, McCollum C. Clinical trial of calcium alginate haemostatic swabs. *Br J Surg* 1990;77(5):568-570.

42. McCarthy PM. Fibrin glue in cardiothoracic surgery. *Transfus Med Rev* 1993;7(3):173-179.

Control of Perioperative Bleeding With Serine Protease Inhibitors

David Royston, MD, FFARCS

Serine protease inhibitors (SERPINs), if correctly investigated and used, can revolutionize future pharmacologic approaches to many medical problems, and not just bleeding. This group of compounds is likely to become recognized as introducing a dramatically new concept in therapy of significant patient benefit. These compounds are important because protease enzymes are essential to the control processes involved in both hemostasis and immunity. These host-defense mechanisms are fundamental to all living organisms; the simple systems used by early life forms having evolved into complex, interrelated pathways and cascades. However, the basic principles remain unchanged, and the human being can be regarded as a primitive two-sided organism surrounded by a membrane that functions to keep the inside in and the outside out.[1]

The mechanisms that operate to prevent the inside from escaping to the outside comprise the hemostatic system; mechanisms that prevent anything recognized as nonself from entering from the outside comprise the anti-inflammatory system. Both systems require some sort of cellular element that can recognize injury and be able to move to the area of injury and adhere there; the movement may occur simply by the flow of intraluminal contents or, in the case of white cells, by active migration. In both systems, a precursor (or zymogen) is required, as is an enzyme that acts to convert the zymogen to its active form. The converting enzyme is always a protease. Virtually all protease enzymes in the plasma are serine proteases, based on the amino acid serine. The human body contains many serine proteases, some of which we still do not fully understand. Naturally, all these control proteins are matched by protein antiproteases, which we call SERPINs.[2]

Plasmin, trypsin, thrombin, kallikrein, and elastase are among the body's serine proteases. Like all serine proteases, these contain an active pocket consisting of glycine-aspartate-serine-glycine. Human SERPINs include antithrombin III (AT-III), α_2-macroglobulin, α_1-antitrypsin, and heparin cofactor II (HC II). Other SERPINs include the naturally occurring polypeptide aprotinin and synthetic agents such as gabexate (FOY), nafamostat (Futhan), and certain chlormethyl ketones.

The inhibitory concentrations of SERPINs differ greatly and also depend on the system used for their determination. For example, the data indicating that trypsin is inhibited by low concentrations of aprotinin are derived from determinations made in test-tube systems, and actual inhibitory concentrations in the body remain unknown.[3] There are also problems related to inhibitory effectiveness due to other factors related to the site of the active center in the molecule. For example, the active site of thrombin is identical to that of trypsin. This would suggest that thrombin will be inhibited by the same low concentration of aprotinin. However, this active pocket is protected by a small overhanging flap. Effective thrombin inhibition with aprotinin thus requires a far higher concentration of aprotinin to achieve a stoichiometric inhibition. Alternately, a molecule designed to get under that flap will require only a low concentration to exert an effect.[4]

The various potential anti-inflammatory actions of aprotinin and other protease inhibitors were the subject of a recent review.[1] This presentation will briefly discuss nafamostat and gabexate use and will then focus largely on the efficacy and safety of aprotinin in inhibiting bleeding in clinical use.

NAFAMOSTAT AND GABEXATE

Nafamostat and gabexate have been used extensively in Japan to prevent bleeding associated with contact activation, either in hemodialysis or in plasmapheresis.[5-9] They also have been used to prevent bleeding during cardiovascular surgery and in patients supported long-term with left ventricular assist devices (LVADs) or other mechanical supports.[10-12] In one study reported in *Circulation* by Murase et al,[13] nafamostat use resulted in a 30% reduction in drainage loss during cardiac surgery. Even more important, transfusion requirements were 8 units of blood and blood products in the control patients and only 2 units of blood and blood products in the nafamostat-treated patients. This is a huge difference in transfusion requirements when compared with the amount of patient blood loss. Patient requirements for blood or blood-product transfusion is the most important end point when evaluating SERPIN efficacy.

APROTININ EFFICACY

High-dose aprotinin, now called the Hammersmith dose, was intended to serve as an anti-inflammatory regimen and was designed to produce a constant plasma concentration throughout a bypass procedure when the times to the start of bypass, total bypass ($\approx$ 60 minutes), and ischemic times ($\approx$ 30 minutes) were relatively short.[14,15] Obvious deficiencies in the regimen is a lack of consideration of variables such as the patient's age, weight, and gender; the type of surgery that may be reflected in the ischemic and bypass times; and any time delay from the start of surgery until the institution of bypass, among others. Nevertheless, this regimen has been widely promoted and has been used in numerous studies of bleeding in primary coronary artery bypass graft (CABG) surgery.[16,17]

Aprotinin differs from other pharmacologic interventions such as the lysine analogue antifibrinolytics in its spectrum of efficacy. An analysis of available data suggests that all the pharmacologic SERPINs produce roughly the same reduction in drain losses in primary CABG surgery when compared with ε-aminocaproic acid (EACA) and tranexamic acid (AMCHA) but more important, far greater decreases in patient transfusion requirements are found with SERPIN therapy than with the lysine analogues (Fig 1).[18] Thus, SERPINs can improve hemostasis and stop bleeding, although they can also inhibit certain processes in the coagulation cascade, which poses one of the major enigmas associated with the mode of action of this group of compounds. In particular, aprotinin has unique benefits in patients having repeat heart surgery and in those with endocarditis.[14,15,19-24] The five studies of aprotinin use in reoperations show a very impressive consistency in the amount of decrease in transfusion requirements (Fig 2).

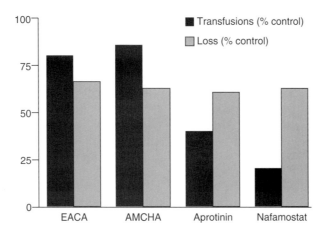

Fig 1. Homologous blood transfusions and drain losses expressed as percentage of control values from studies of various pharmacologic interventions in primary open heart surgery patients. The data show that all agents reduce drain losses, but the serine protease inhibitors aprotinin and nafamostat have a much greater effect in reducing the need for blood transfusions. EACA, ε-aminocaproic acid; AMCHA, tranexamic acid. Reprinted with permission from *International Anesthesiology Clinics,* 1995;33:1550179 fig 1.

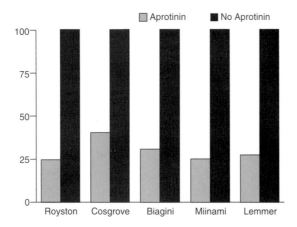

Fig 2. Blood product transfusions from five studies of aprotinin use in patients having reoperation coronary artery bypass surgery.[19-23] Values are normalized to give 100% to the control (no aprotinin) patients. The data show remarkable similarity of effect among centers and countries. Reprinted with permission from *International Anesthesiology Clinics,* 1995;33:1550179 fig 2.

In addition, aprotinin has been found to be beneficial in patients with end-stage cardiopulmonary failure who need heart, lung, or heart-lung transplantation or who may require extracorporeal respiratory support or the insertion of an LVAD.[25-31]

The distinctive efficacy profile of the SERPINs can be also appreciated when considering studies where aprotinin has been directly compared with other agents. In these studies, high-dose aprotinin therapy has been shown to be significantly superior to mechanical blood-conservation techniques such as the use of predonated blood or platelet concentrates.[32,33]

In comparison with other pharmacologic agents, high-dose aprotinin is significantly more effective than high-dose AMCHA in patients having primary CABG surgery.[34]

Two important points about aprotinin efficacy emerged from one of the studies of aprotinin in reoperation patients.[20] The data indicate a dose-response relationship with regard to drain losses: The administration of half the Hammersmith dose still resulted in a significant reduction of drain losses, although not as large a reduction as with the full dose. However, this was not the case with blood-transfusion requirements. Patients who received the half dose were still exposed to roughly 10 units of donor blood and blood products, while patients who received the full dose required the transfusion of only about 4 units of blood and blood products (Fig 3). It should be noted that in this study (conducted at the Cleveland Clinic) both control and aprotinin-treated patients also benefited from many additional efforts directed at preventing blood loss, including hemodilution, cell salvage, reinfusion of shed blood, and if physicians thought it necessary, administration of desmopressin or EACA. Nevertheless, high-dose aprotinin still produced a profound benefit in these patients, something no other agent has been shown to do.

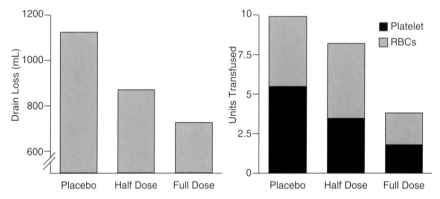

Fig 3. Drain losses and blood-product transfusion requirements with aprotinin treatment. Redrawn from data in reference 20. A dose-response relationship existed with regard to drain losses, but this was not the case with blood transfusion requirements. Patients who received the half-dose were still exposed to roughly 10 units of donor blood and blood products (not significantly different from placebo), while patients who received the full dose required the transfusion of only about 4 units of blood and blood products. This difference between half-dose and full-dose aprotinin was statistically significant.

Aprotinin also has been shown to be effective in patients with thrombocytopenia, in patients who received aspirin preoperatively, after fibrinolytic therapy, and in the presence of other agents, such as ticlopidine or clopidogrel known to increase bleeding tendency by inhibition of platelet functions.[35-41] In contrast, a number of studies have failed to show any effectiveness for lysine analogues in the presence of thrombocytopenia.[42]

Aprotinin additionally has been shown to be effective in a variety of other surgeries; for example, hip-replacement surgery.[43,44] The most recent study from Belgium show that aprotinin resulted in a small reduction in drain losses but a large reduction in transfusion requirements.[45] The effect of aprotinin was found to be even greater in a study of hip-replacement surgery in patients with septic arthritis at the time of their surgery. Such data certainly confound the view long held by many that aprotinin would only be effective in cardiac surgery because its action involved the prevention of contact activation in some way, but they also highlight questions about how the drug really works and what else we still do not know about it.

A number of studies[46-53] (although by no means all[54]) have shown that aprotinin results in a large reduction in the amount of blood products required during liver transplantation. The reduction in blood-product use was associated with significant reductions in times on ventilation and times in the intensive care unit (ICU), both of which have cost consequences in hospital practice.[50,51]

Aprotinin has been used in obstetrics and gynecology, reducing bleeding and the need for cesarean section after *abruptio placentae* and preventing bleeding associated with consumptive coagulopathy in patients with amniotic fluid embolus or dead-fetus syndrome.[55-58] Aprotinin also has been used in neurosurgery, preventing oozing and decreasing rebleeding more effectively than hydrogen peroxide in tumors of the meninges, which may be a tissue plasminogen activator (t-PA) related phenomenon and reducing the rebleeding rate in subarachnoid hemorrhage.[59-62] In addition, reduced perioperative bleeding has been associated with aprotinin treatment in vascular and genitourinary surgery.[63-65]

Aprotinin has been viewed by some as an antiplatelet agent, somehow able to protect platelet functions. In a study of aprotinin use to prevent deep-vein thrombosis (DVT) in orthopedic surgery, aprotinin was shown to prevent the normal tendency of platelets to become more adherent to glass beads.[66,67] A more recent study also looked at the effect of aprotinin on platelet function; in this case, the aggregation of platelets induced by the addition of adenosine diphosphate (ADP).[34] Platelet reactivity to ADP normally decreases during surgery. Patients undergoing primary CABG surgery were given either high-dose AMCHA or high-dose aprotinin. Aprotinin significantly reduced bleeding, while AMCHA did not. However, the decrease in aggregation to ADP normally associated with the surgery was almost fully reversed by AMCHA but less so by aprotinin. Thus, a lysine analogue showed a greater effect than aprotinin in this particular test of platelet function, although it did not at all modify bleeding. Analysis of the data obtained in this study shows no real differences in the effects of the two pharmacologic interventions on protein C, D-dimers, AT-III, or prothrombin F1+2, emphasizing the difficulty in understanding precisely the mechanisms of action of these compounds. However, these puzzling data may largely be due to the fact that the blood samples being analyzed are taken from large peripheral veins and, therefore, the findings may have no relationship to what is actually happening at the tissue level.

Another enigma of aprotinin's mechanism of action was demonstrated in an animal model of pure fibrinolytic bleeding. In this study, modest doses of aprotinin (ie, about one-quarter of the dose given to a human during bypass surgery) reversed the bleeding tendency.[68] The use of AMCHA or lysine analogues, although they are antifibrinolytics, did not stop the bleeding associated with fibrinolysis.

APROTININ SAFETY

Concern that aprotinin might cause graft occlusion originated essentially with the Cleveland Clinic report of some deaths in their reoperation series.[20] A portion of those patients who went to postmortem examination showed graft occlusion. In fact, only 6 out of 522 grafts were occluded, but since they all appeared in the half-dose aprotinin group, these graft thromboses were attributed to aprotinin. I have argued previously, and on theoretical grounds only, that there may be a potential for increased thrombotic risk with lower doses of aprotinin or of the lysine antifibrinolytics.[69] Indeed, another study showed that EACA does not cause a hypercoagulable state,[70] but the published report of this study included surgeon observations of more clot formation during takedown of the internal mammary artery and more observed clots after cardiopulmonary bypass in the EACA-treated group.

A number of different studies have provided aprotinin safety data. A single-center study done in Munich of morbidity and mortality in patients having both valve and CABG surgery showed no difference in mortality between 882 control patients and 902 patients treated with aprotinin.[71] A United Kingdom open study of 671 patients treated with aprotinin, among whom 457 patients were undergoing reoperations and 79 had endocarditis, reported only 13 instances of adverse effects: 4 were allergic reactions, 7 involved renal impairment, and only 2 involved thrombosis.[24] Of the 2 reported cases of thrombosis, 1 involved a patient's vein grafts, and the surgeons admitted that a technical problem was probably responsible. The other thrombosis occurred in an oxygenator primed with blood and recirculating for 6 hours prior to surgery, during which time the pump failed. Finally, a report of the use of high-dose aprotinin therapy in 2190 patients treated in one center in Europe failed to show any deleterious effects related to thrombotic events.[72]

Four studies that were focused specifically on graft patency with aprotinin use found no significant difference in the frequency of graft occlusion between control and aprotinin-treated patients, with an approximately 6% frequency of occlusion.[21,73-75] Three studies reporting the incidence of myocardial infarctions showed myocardial infarctions occurring in about 8% of control patients and about 11% of aprotinin-treated patients.[20,21,38] For comparison, two recently reported large studies comparing results in patients undergoing angioplasty and patients undergoing CABG showed a Q-wave myocardial infarction rate of approximately 8% to 10% in patients who had surgery,[76,77] basically no different from the myocardial infarction rate found in the aprotinin groups in the studies cited above. In two studies of aprotinin use in hip surgery, patients treated with aprotinin failed to show any evidence of DVT.[45,78]

The accumulated data on aprotinin safety lead me to conclude that this drug does not increase thrombotic risk.

SOME QUESTIONS ABOUT HEPARIN AND APROTININ

The three places in our bodies where the inside meets the outside are the skin, the lungs, and the gut, and it is at these sites that mast cells are found. Mast cells contain both heparin and aprotinin. Heparin acts as an anticoagulant, modifying AT-III and, probably more important, stimulating release of tissue factor pathway inhibitor. Heparin also acts as a significant immune modulator, causing immunosuppression. For example, heparin will inhibit wheal formation after dermal injection of histamine and complement fragments in human. Heparin is also an inhibitor of smooth-muscle migration and proliferation. We must wonder whether heparin is in the body to act primarily as an anticoagulant or whether it is there for some other reason.

Aprotinin is not present until after birth and, therefore, cannot be fundamental; it appears after birth only when an immune process is required. Aprotinin is found in many lower orders of life, including anemones and crustaceans. Why is it there? Does it serve some fundamentally important purpose in these animals? Aprotinin is found in both native and modified forms in many species: It is an anticoagulant and an anti-infective; it is used in many species to block potassium channels and/or calcium channels; and it serves as a neurotoxin in certain spiders and snakes. So what, in fact, do we use aprotinin for?

References

1. Royston D. *International Journal of Cardiology* 1996. In press.

2. Laskowski M, Kato I. Protein inhibitors of proteinases. *Ann Rev Biochem* 1980;49:593-626.

3. Fritz H, Wunderer G. Biochemistry and applications of aprotinin, the kallikrein inhibitor from bovine organs. *Arzneimittelforschung* 1983;33:479-494.

4. Tapparelli C, Metternich R, Ehrhardt C, Cook NS. Synthetic low-molecular-weight thrombin inhibitors: molecular design and pharmacological profile. *Trends Pharmacol Sci* 1993;14:366-376.

5. Taenaka N, Shimada Y, Hirata T, Nishijima M, Yoshiya I. New approach to regional anticoagulation in hemodialysis using gabexate mesilate (FOY). *Crit Care Med* 1982;10:773-775.

6. Taenaka N, Terada N, Takahashi H, et al. Hemodialysis using gabexate mesilate (FOY) in patients with a high bleeding risk. *Crit Care Med* 1986;14:481-483.

7. Matsuo T, Kario K, Nakao K, Yamada T, Matsuo M. Anticoagulation with nafamostat mesilate, a synthetic protease inhibitor, in hemodialysis patients with a bleeding risk. *Haemostasis* 1993;23:135-141.

8. Hosokawa S, Oyamaguchi A, Yoshida O. Clinical evaluation of nafamostat mesilate (FUT 175): a new anticoagulant for plasmapheresis. *ASAIO J Trans* 1992;38:59-60.

9. Kinugasa E, Akizawa T, Nakashima Y, Wakasa M, Koshikawa S. Nafamostat as anticoagulant for membrane plasmapheresis in high bleeding risk patients. *Int J Artif Organs* 1992;15:595-600.

10. Okamoto T, Chung YK, Choi H, Terasaki H, Morioka T. Experimental results using nafamostat mesilate as anticoagulant during extracorporeal lung assist for 24 hours in dogs. *Artif Organs* 1993;17:30-36.

11. Takahama T, Kanai F, Hiraishi M, et al. Application of a prostacyclin analogue (PG) and protease inhibitor (FUT) as anticoagulants with an LVAD system. *ASAIO Trans* 1986;32:253-257.

12. Takahama T, Kanai F, Hiraishi M, et al. Comparative study of anticoagulation therapy with an LVAD system. *ASAIO Trans* 1987;33:227-234.

13. Murase M, Usui A, Tomita Y, Maeda M, Koyama T, Abe T. Nafamostat mesilate reduces blood loss during open heart surgery. *Circulation* 1993;88:432-436.

14. Royston D. The serine antiprotease aprotinin (Trasylol): a novel approach to reducing postoperative bleeding. *Blood Coag Fibrinolys* 1990;1:55-69.

15. Bidstrup BP, Royston D, Sapsford RN, Taylor KM. Reduction in blood loss and blood use after cardiopulmonary bypass with high-dose aprotinin (Trasylol). *J Thorac Cardiovasc Surg* 1989;97:364-72.

16. Davis R, Whittington R. Aprotinin: a review of its pharmacology and therapeutic efficacy in reducing blood loss associated with cardiac surgery. *Drugs* 1995;49:954-983.

17. Royston D. High-dose aprotinin therapy: a review of the first five years' experience. *J Cardiothorac Vasc Anesth* 1992;6:76-100.

18. Royston D. Blood-sparing drugs: aprotinin, tranexamic acid and ε-aminocaproic acid. In: Feeley TW, Royston D, eds. *International Anesthesiology Clinics*. Boston, Mass: Little, Brown and Company; 1995; 33:155-179.

19. Biagini A, Comite C, Russo V. High dose aprotinin to reduce blood loss in patients undergoing redo open heart surgery. *Acta Anaesthesiol Belg* 1992;43:181-186.

20. Cosgrove DM, Heric B, Lytle BW, et al. Aprotinin therapy for reoperative myocardial revascularization: a placebo-controlled study. *Ann Thorac Surg* 1992;54:1031-1036.

21. Lemmer JH Jr, Stanford W, Bonney SL, et al. Aprotinin for coronary bypass operations: efficacy, safety, and influence on early saphenous vein graft patency: a multicenter, randomized, double-blind, placebo-controlled study. *J Thorac Cardiovasc Surg* 1994;107:543-551.

22. Minami K, Notohamiprodjo G, Buschler H, Prohaska W, Reichelt W, Korfer R. Alpha-2 plasmin inhibitor-plasmin complex and postoperative blood loss: double-blind study with aprotinin in reoperation for myocardial revascularization. *J Thorac Cardiovasc Surg* 1993;106:934-936. Letter.

23. Royston D, Bidstrup BP, Taylor KM, Sapsford RN. Effect of aprotinin on need for blood transfusion after repeat open-heart surgery. *Lancet* 1987;2:1289-1291.

24. Bidstrup BP, Harrison J, Royston D, Taylor KM, Treasure T. Aprotinin therapy in cardiac operations: a report on use in 41 cardiac centers in the United Kingdom. *Ann Thorac Surg* 1993;55:971-976.

25. Havel M, Owen AN, Simon P, et al. Decreasing use of donated blood and reduction of bleeding after orthotopic heart transplantation by use of aprotinin. *J Heart Lung Transplant* 1992;11:348-349.

26. Peterson KL, DeCampli WM, Feeley TW, Starnes VA. Blood loss and transfusion requirements in cystic fibrosis patients undergoing heart-lung or lung transplantation. *J Cardiothorac Vasc Anesth* 1995;9:59-62.

27. Kesten S, de Hoyas A, Chaparro C, Westney G, Winton T, Maurer JR. Aprotinin reduces blood loss in lung transplant recipients. *Ann Thorac Surg* 1995;59:877-879.

28. Propst JW, Siegel LC, Feeley TW. Effect of aprotinin on transfusion requirements during repeat sternotomy for cardiac transplantation surgery. *Transplant Proc* 1994;26:3719-3721.

29. Royston D. Aprotinin therapy in heart and heart-lung transplantation. *J Heart Lung Transplant* 1993;12:S19-25.

30. Brunet F, Mira JP, Belghith M, et al. Effects of aprotinin on hemorrhagic complications in ARDS patients during prolonged extracorporeal CO_2 removal. *Intensive Care Med* 1992;18:364-367.

31. Goldstein D, Selmonridge J, Chen J, et al. Use of aprotinin in LVAD recipients reduces blood loss, blood use and perioperative mortality. *Ann Thorac Surg* 1995;59:1063-1068.

32. Vedrinne C, Girard C, Jegaden O, et al. Reduction in blood loss and blood use after cardiopulmonary bypass with high-dose aprotinin versus autologous fresh whole blood transfusion. *J Cardiothorac Vasc Anesth* 1992;6:319-323.

33. Shinfeld A, Zippel D, Lavee J, et al. Aprotinin improves hemostasis after cardiopulmonary bypass better than single-donor platelet concentrate. *Ann Thorac Surg* 1995;59:872-876.

34. Blauhut B, Harringer W, Bettelheim P, Doran JE, Spath P, Lundsgaard-Hansen P. Comparison of the effects of aprotinin and tranexamic acid on blood loss and related variables after cardiopulmonary bypass. *J Thorac Cardiovasc Surg* 1994;108:1083-1091.

35. Deviri E, Izhar U, Drenger B, Glick Y, Borman JB. Aprotinin treatment during open heart operation in a patient with severe thrombocytopenia. *Ann Thorac Surg* 1992;54:1018-1019. Letter.

36. Roath OS, Majer RV, Smith AG. The use of aprotinin in thrombocytopenic patients: a preliminary evaluation. *Blood Coag Fibrinolys* 1990;1:235-237.

37. Bidstrup B, Royston D, McGuiness C, Sapsford R. Aprotinin in aspirin -pretreated patients. *Perfusion* 1990;5:77-81.

38. Murkin JM, Lux J, Shannon NA, et al. Aprotinin significantly decreases bleeding and transfusion requirements in patients receiving aspirin and undergoing cardiac operations. *J Thorac Cardiovasc Surg* 1994;107:554-561.

39. Akhtar TM, Goodchild CS, Boylan MK. Reversal of streptokinase-induced bleeding with aprotinin for emergency cardiac surgery. *Anaesthesia* 1992;47:226-228.

40. Efstratiadis T, Munsch C, Crossman D, Taylor K. Aprotinin use in emergency coronary operation after streptokinase treatment. *Ann Thorac Surg* 1991;52:1320-1321. Comments.

41. Herbert JM, Bernat A, Maffrand JP. Aprotinin reduces clopidogrel-induced prolongation of the bleeding time in the rat. *Thromb Res* 1993;71:433-441.

42. Fricke W, Alling D, Kimball J, Griffith P, Klein H. Lack of efficacy of tranexamic acid in thrombocytopenic bleeding. *Transfusion* 1991;31:345-348.

43. Wollinsky KH, Mehrkens HH, Freytag T, Geiger P, Weindler M. [Does aprotinin lessen intraoperative blood loss?]. *Anasth Intensivmed Notfallmed Schmerzther* 1991;26:208-210.

44. Haas S, Fritsche H, Ritter H, et al. Fuhrt eine perioperative gabe des plasmainhibitors aprotinin zu einer steigerung des postoperativen thromboserisikos? In: Hartel W, Bager H, Ungeheuer, eds. *Chirurgisches Forum '91, f. experim. u klinische Forschubg.* Berlin, Germany: Springer-Verlag; 1991:371-374.

45. Janssens M, Joris J, David JL, Lemaire R, Lamy M. High-dose aprotinin reduces blood loss in patients undergoing total hip replacement surgery. *Anesthesiology* 1994;80:23-29. Comments.

46. Bechstein WO, Riess H, Blumhardt G, et al. Aprotinin in orthotopic liver transplantation. *Semin Thromb Hemost* 1993;19:262-267.

47. Gerlach H, Rossaint R, Slama K, et al. No requirement for cryoprecipitate or platelet transfusion during liver transplantation. *Transplant Proc* 1993;25:1813-1816.

48. Grosse H, Lobbes W, Frambach M, Ringe B, Barthels M. Influence of high-dose aprotinin on hemostasis and blood requirement in orthotopic liver transplantation. *Semin Thromb Hemost* 1993;19:302-305.

49. Ickx B, Pradier O, DeGroote F, et al. Effect of two different dosages of aprotonin on perioperative blood loss during liver transplantation. *Semin Thromb Hemost* 1993;19:300-301.

50. Mallett S, Rolles K, Cox D, Burroughs A, Hunt B. Intraoperative use of aprotinin (Trasylol) in orthotopic liver transplantation. *Transplant Proc* 1991;23:1931-1932.

51. Mallett SV, Alcock R, Cox D, Davidson B, Rolles K. Aprotinin and orthotopic liver transplantation. *Lancet* 1992;340:493.

52. Smith O, Hazlehurst G, Brozovic B, et al. Impact of aprotinin on blood transfusion requirements in liver transplantation. *Transfus Med* 1993;3:97-102.

53. Suarez M, Sangro B, Herrero JI, et al. Effectiveness of aprotinin in orthotopic liver transplantation. *Semin Thromb Hemost* 1993;19:292-296.

54. Groh J, Welte M, Azad SC, Anthuber M, Haller M, Kratzer MA. Does aprotinin really reduce blood loss in orthotopic liver transplantation? *Semin Thromb Hemost* 1993;19:306-308.

55. Sher G. Trasylol in the management of *abruptio placentae* with consumption coagulopathy and uterine inertia. *J Reprod Med* 1980;25:113-118.

56. Sher G, Statland BE. *Abruptio placentae* with coagulopathy: a rational basis for management. *Clin Obstet Gynecol* 1985;28:15-23.

57. Oney T, Schander K, Muller N, Fromm G, Lang N. [Amniotic fluid embolism with coagulation disorder—a case report (author's trans)]. *Geburtshilfe Frauenheilkd* 1982;42:25-28.

58. Suzuki S, Kanagawa Y. [Treatment of obstetric disseminated intravascular coagulation]. *Rinsho Ketsueki* 1982;23:827-835.

59. Tzonos T, Giromini D. Aprotinin for intraoperative haemostasis. *Neurosurg Rev* 1981;4:193-194.

60. Palmer JD, Francis DA, Roath OS, Francis JL, Iannotti F. Hyperfibrinolysis during intracranial surgery: effect of high-dose aprotinin. *J Neurol Neurosurg Psychiatry* 1995;58:104-106.

61. Guidetti B, Spallone A. The role of antifibrinolytic therapy in the preoperative management of recently ruptured intracranial aneurysms. *Surg Neurol* 1981;15:239-248.

62. Spallone A. Antifibrinolytics in aneurysmal subarachnoid haemorrhage: a retrospective comparison of two different forms of antifibrinolytic therapy. *Acta Neurochir Wien* 1982;63:245-250.

63. Lord RA, Roath OS, Thompson JF, Chant AD, Francis JL. Effect of aprotinin on neutrophil function after major vascular surgery. *Br J Surg* 1992;79:517-521.

64. Thompson J, Roath OS, Francis J, Webster J, Chant A. Aprotinin in peripheral vascular surgery. *Lancet* 1990;335:911.

65. Schmutzler R, Furstenberg H. [Fibrinolysis and loss of blood following prostatic surgery and their susceptibility to antifibrinolytics: epsilon-aminocaproic acid and the kallikrein inhibitor Trasylol]. *Dtsch Med Wochenschr* 1966;91:297-303.

66. Ketterl R, Haas S, Lechner F. Wirkung von Aprotinin auf die Thrombo- zytenfunktion währen Hüft-Totalendoprosthesenoperation. *Med Welt* 1980;31: 1239 -1241.

67. Ketterl R, Haas S, Heiss A. Zur Wirkung des natürlichen Proteinasen inhibitors Aprotinin auf die Plättchenfunktion beim alloarthroplastischen Hüftgelenkersatz. *Med Welt* 1982;33:480-486.

68. de-Bono DP, Pringle S, Underwood I. Differential effects of aprotinin and tranexamic acid on cerebral bleeding and cutaneous bleeding time during rt-PA infusion. *Thromb Res* 1991;61:159-163.

69. Royston D. Intraoperative coronary thrombosis: can aprotinin be incriminated? *J Cardiothorac Vasc Anesth* 1994;8:137-141. Editorial; Comment.

70. Arom KV, Emery RW. Decreased postoperative drainage with addition of epsilon- aminocaproic acid before cardiopulmonary bypass. *Ann Thorac Surg* 1994;57:1108- 1112.

71. Dietrich D, Barankay A, Hahnel C, Richter J. High dose aprotinin in cardiac surgery: three years' experience in 1784 patients. *J Cardiothorac Vasc Anesth* 1992;6:936-941.

72. Paroli A, Antona C, Gerometta P, et al. The effect of high dose aprotinin and other factors on bleeding and revisions for bleeding in adult coronary and valve operations: an analysis of 2190 patients during a five-year period (1987-1991). *Eur J Cardiothorac Surg* 1995;9:77-82.

73. Bidstrup BP, Underwood SR, Sapsford RN, Streets EM. Effect of aprotinin (Trasylol) on aortacoronary bypass graft patency. *J Thorac Cardiovasc Surg* 1993;105:147-152.

74. Havel M, Grabenwoger F, Schneider J, et al. Aprotinin does not decrease early graft patency after coronary artery bypass grafting despite reducing postoperative bleeding and use of donated blood. *J Thorac Cardiovasc Surg* 1994;107:807-810.

75. Lass M, Welz A, Kochs M, Mayer G, Schwandt M, Hannekum A. Aprotinin in elective primary bypass surgery: graft patency and clinical efficacy. *Eur J Cardiothorac Surg* 1995;9:206-210.

76. King SB 3rd, Lembo NJ, Weintraub WS, et al. A randomized trial comparing coronary angioplasty with coronary bypass surgery: Emory Angioplasty versus Surgery Trial (EAST). *N Engl J Med* 1994;331:1044-1050. Comments.

77. Hamm CW, Reimers J, Ischinger T, Rupprecht HJ, Berger J, Bleifeld W. A randomized study of coronary angioplasty compared with bypass surgery in patients with symptomatic multivessel coronary disease: German Angioplasty Bypass Surgery Investigation (GABI). *N Engl J Med* 1994;331:1037-1043.

78. Murkin JM, Shannon NA, Bourne RB, Rorabeck CH, Cruickshank M, Wyile G. Aprotinin decreases blood loss in patients undergoing revision or bilateral total hip arthroplasty. *Anesth Analg* 1995;80:343-348.

Workshop I:
Blood Conservation in
Orthopedic Surgery

The Bleeding Problem in Orthopedic Surgery

Michael G. Neuwirth, MD

The risk of significant perioperative blood loss is associated with many orthopedic procedures, including elective procedures such as total-hip or total-knee replacement, complex shoulder surgery, complex spinal reconstructive procedures, and trauma. This presentation will focus on elective orthopedic surgery.

The goal of the orthopedic surgical team should be to reduce perioperative blood loss to a level that would hopefully eliminate homologous blood use in the elective orthopedic population. The risks of blood transfusion must be balanced against its benefits.

RISKS OF HOMOLOGOUS BLOOD-PRODUCT TRANSFUSION

The transmission of infection, eg, human immunodeficiency virus (HIV), human T cell lymphotropic virus (HTLV-1), hepatitis B and C, remains a major risk associated with transfusion of homologous blood products. However, improved testing procedures have reduced the risk of HIV and hepatitis infection. Data cited elsewhere in this book report the risk of HIV infection as being approximately one case per 225,000 units transfused and the risk of posttransfusion hepatitis as 1 in 3300 units (Klein. The Risk of Perioperative Transfusion). Risks still remain for infection from other viral organisms, protozoa, parasites, and emerging new organisms. Although the risk of infection from homologous blood is small, the public perception that blood transfusions are associated with transmission of disease, in particular HIV, makes this a significant problem for the clinician.

Other risks associated with blood-component administration include transfusion reactions that range from a fairly high incidence of fever, chills, and urticaria to a rare incidence of severe acute reactions due to major blood-group incompatibility or bacterial contamination of the blood component.[1-3] Longer-term immunologic effects may be associated with the development of antibodies to blood cells and the possible increased susceptibility to perioperative bacterial infections.[4,5] Increased risk of cancer recurrence after cancer surgery have been reported.[6,7]

Data from the American National Red Cross Blood Bank show that a significant number of blood products have to be recalled after having been released as safe for patient use. One major reason for recall is a donor history of HIV or hepatitis infection despite a negative lab test for these infectious agents.

BENEFITS OF BLOOD-PRODUCT TRANSFUSION

Blood transfusion should be considered if the patient's oxygen transfer to the tissues is compromised due to anemia, and/or if clotting factors and platelets are needed to restore hemostasis. Indications for blood-product transfusion must be considered on an individual patient basis. The rule that a hematocrit below 30% is the indication for transfusion no longer applies, and patients with normal cardiac function can compensate with hematocrits as low as 10% to 15%.

REDUCED-BLEEDING TECHNIQUES AND
ALTERNATIVES TO HOMOLOGOUS BLOOD

It is axiomatic that meticulous surgical hemostasis will have a significant effect on perioperative bleeding. Other techniques can be applied to orthopedic surgery, including induced hypotension and the proper positioning of the patient.[8-12] There are several alternatives to homologous blood transfusion. These include: autologous predonation, acute hemodilution, use of erythropoetin, intraoperative blood salvage, and the use of pharmacologic agents such as desmopressin or aprotinin.[8,13-20]

Each surgical team should develop a strategy to reduce perioperative blood loss and minimize homologous blood use in elective orthopedic surgery. This should include patient and surgical team education, with complete discussion of the risks and benefits associated with the use of homologous blood. The patient should give informed consent. Appropriate preoperative evaluation of the patient's likely needs for transfusion should be carried out.

A recent survey undertaken at the Hospital for Joint Diseases, Orthopedic Institute emphasizes how a comprehensive approach to blood conservation can have significant results in limiting the use of homologous blood. In this series of 109 patients undergoing circumferential spinal fusion, the blood loss ranged from 400 mL to 4200 mL, with an average loss of 1400 mL. However, despite these substantial losses, the use of other techniques of blood conservation, predonation of autologous blood and intraoperative salvage, resulted in only 3 out of these 109 patients requiring homologous blood transfusion (unpublished data).

REFERENCES

1. Murphy WG, McClelland DB. Deceptively low morbidity from failure to practice safe blood transfusion: an analysis of serious blood transfusion errors. *Vox Sang* 1989;57:59-62.

2. Linden JV, Paul B, Dressler KP. A report of 104 transfusion errors in New York State. *Transfusion* 1992;32:601-606.

3. Contreras M, Mollison PL. ABC of transfusion: immunological complications of transfusion. *Br Med J* 1990;300:173-176.

4. NIH Consensus Development Summaries. Fresh-frozen plasma: indications and risks. *Conn Med* 1985;49:295-297.

5. Blumberg N, Heal JM. Transfusion-induced immunomodulation and its possible role in cancer recurrence and perioperative bacterial infection. *Yale J Biol Med* 1990;63:429-433.

6. Chesi R, Borghi B, Lari S. Perioperative blood transfusions and survival in osteosarcoma. *Cancer Treat Res* 1993;62:25-28.

7. Chung M, Steinmetz OK, Gordon PH. Perioperative blood transfusion and outcome after resection for colorectal carcinoma. *Br J Surg* 1993;80:427-432. Comments.

8. Solomon DE. Induced hypotension and isovolemic hemodilution. *Spine* 1991;5:1.

9. Lam AM. Induced hypotension. *Can Anaesth Soc J* 1984;31:S56-62.

10. Sivarajan M, Amory DW, Everett GB, Buffington C. Blood pressure, not cardiac output, determines blood loss during induced hypotension. *Anesth Analg* 1980;59:203-206.

11. Phillips WA, Hensinger RN. Control of blood loss during scoliosis surgery. *Clin Orthop* 1988;229:88-93.

12. DiStefano VJ, Klein KS, Nixon JE, Andrews ET. Intra-operative analysis of the effects of position and body habitus on surgery of the low back: a preliminary report. *Clin Orthop* 1974;99:51-56.

13. Goodnough LT, Shafron D, Marcus RE. The impact of preoperative autologous blood donation on orthopaedic surgical practice. *Vox Sang* 1990;59:65-69.

14. MacEwen GD, Bennett E, Guille JT. Autologous blood transfusions in children and young adults with low body weight undergoing spinal surgery. *J Pediatr Orthop* 1990;10:750-753.

15. Canadian Orthopedic Perioperative Erythropoietin Study Group. Effectiveness of perioperative recombinant human erythropoietin in elective hip replacement. *Lancet* 1993;341:1227-1232.

16. Bernstein D, Rosenberg AD, Blackshear C. Intraoperative cell salvage in orthopedic surgery. *Anesth Analg* 1994;78:S37.

17. Salzman EW, Weinstein MJ, Reilly D, Ware JA. Adventures in hemostasis: desmopressin in cardiac surgery. *Arch Surg* 1993;128:212-217.

18. Temeck BK, Bachenheimer LC, Katz NM, Coughlin SS, Wallace RB. Desmo-pressin acetate in cardiac surgery: a double-blind, randomized study. *South Med J* 1994;87:611-615.

19. Murkin JM, Shannon NA, Bourne RB, Rorabeck CH, Cruickshank M, Wyile G. Aprotinin decreases blood loss in patients undergoing revision or bilateral total hip arthroplasty. *Anesth Analg* 1995;80:343-348.

20. Janssens M, Joris J, David JL, Lemaire R, Lamy M. High-dose aprotinin reduces blood loss in patients undergoing total hip replacement surgery. *Anesthesiology* 1994;80:23-29.

Methods to Avoid Homologous Transfusion in Orthopedic Surgery

Andrew D. Rosenberg, MD

Patients undergoing elective orthopedic surgery commonly ask how to avoid receiving blood products from someone else. They are concerned about possible transmission of infectious diseases such as the human immunodeficiency virus (HIV), hepatitis, and cytomegalovirus (CMV). Transfusion-related complications and allergic reactions are also a concern. In orthopedic surgery, there is concern that homologous blood transfusion may increase the incidence of postoperative infection.[1] A number of methods, used either individually or in combination, can be employed to avoid homologous transfusion:

- *Autologous predonation.* Patient predonates blood at intervals starting 30 to 35 days preoperatively.

- *Normovolemic hemodilution.* Blood is drawn from the patient in the operating room prior to incision and normovolemia is maintained with crystalloid or colloid.

- *Intraoperative blood salvage.* Blood ordinarily lost during surgery is salvaged, washed, and reinfused.

- *Postoperative blood salvage.* Wound drainage is reinfused into the patient.

- *Surgical and anesthetic techniques.* These include patient positioning and medications to decrease bleeding.

- *Transfusion-trigger alterations.* Transfusion-trigger guidelines of 10 gm/dL or hematocrit of 30% need not be adhered to; instead, physiologic needs specific to each patient should determine course of action.

Autologous Predonation

Predonation should be available to patients who have hemoglobin levels above 11 g/dL.[2] Of interest is that elderly patients have fewer reactions during predonation than younger patients.[3] Patients who have unstable angina or severe aortic stenosis cannot predonate; however, patients undergoing cardiac and vascular surgery can donate if time permits.[4] Patients who weigh less than 110 pounds can predonate partial units. A study by MacEwen shows the effectiveness of this in children scheduled for scoliosis surgery.[5] The volume of blood taken was based on body weight (less than 100 pounds). An average of 811 mL of blood was collected in multiple predonations. Sixty-three percent of the patients did not receive homologous blood, and the remaining 37% had a reduced need for donor blood.

Risks of Preoperative Autologous Donation

The risks of autologous donations are not significantly different from blood-bank donations. Generally, these involve vasovagal reactions, with a 3% incidence of lightheadedness, a 0.3% incidence of transient loss of consciousness, and a 0.03% incidence of self-limited seizures.[4]

Patients at risk from predonating blood include first-time donors, women, patients of low body weight, and anyone who has had a previous reaction.

Autologous predonators are not at any higher risk of significant, moderate, or mild reactions than homologous donors, as noted in a study by McVay.[3]

Patients who predonate are commonly given iron supplementation. Goodnough has demonstrated that erythropoietin (EPO) may also be advantageous in patients who have to donate multiple units.[6] Erythropoietin is produced by the kidney and is a regulator of erythropoiesis. It interacts with receptors in the bone marrow to enhance erythroid proliferation and maturation, with resultant increased red blood cell (RBC) production. In this study, he demonstrated that patients who received EPO were able to donate more units than those who just received iron and a placebo. The RBC mass in the donated blood of the patients who received EPO was 41% higher than the patients who did not receive EPO. This treatment should be of value for patients required to donate up to 6 units preoperatively but may not be necessary for those requiring predonation of only 2 to 3 units.

The endogenous EPO production in response to phlebotomy is short-lived, and the sustained levels obtained with exogenous erythropoietin cannot be achieved.[7]

Recommendations for Predonation
At the Hospital for Joint Diseases, we recommend that our total hip-replacement patients predonate 2 units prior to surgery. When combined with other salvage techniques such as intraoperative cell salvage and reinfusion devices in the recovery room, this decreases the risk of receiving a homologous transfusion, and only 4% of patients undergoing total hip replacement require homologous transfusions. Patients scheduled for spine surgery commonly donate 3 or more units.

Normovolemic Hemodilution
The underlying concept of normovolemic hemodilution is the minimizing of RBC loss if the patient bleeds during surgery. A 1-liter blood loss with a hematocrit of 45% equates to 450 mL of RBCs. A 1-liter blood loss if the patient has been hemodiluted to a hematocrit of 25% reduces the RBC loss to 250 mL. RBCs removed preoperatively can then be reinfused postoperatively. This process may be summarized as follows:

After the patient is anesthetized, blood is drawn and colloid or crystalloid is simultaneously administered to maintain normovolemia. The following formula determines the amount of blood that can be drawn:

$$\text{Amount to be drawn} = \frac{\text{EBV} \times \{\text{Ho} - \text{Ht}\}}{\left(\dfrac{\text{Ho} + \text{Ht}}{2}\right)}$$

EBV =   Estimated blood volume

Ho =   Starting Hct

Ht =   Target Hct

Since the blood donation bags at our institution will handle 450 mL of blood and an appropriate amount of anticoagulant (63 mL) has already been added to the bag, blood must be drawn in unit amounts of 450 mL. If less than 450 mL, of blood is collected, the bag will contain too much anticoagulant; if more than 450 mL, the amount of anticoagulant will be insufficient for the blood collected. Special care must be taken to ensure that regular transfusion bags are not used in children unless 450 mL is to be withdrawn. Not taking this precaution may result in too much anticoagulant being administered systemically when the blood is reinfused. After the patient is asleep, blood is drawn via gravity. Care has to be taken to gently rock the blood back and forth, which will allow the anticoagulant to mix. The transfusion bag is placed on a scale, and the scale has to be calibrated (rezeroed) to take the weight of the blood bag and anticoagulant into effect. As blood is drawn, fluid is reinfused as either crystalloid in a 3:1 ratio or colloid in a 2:1 ratio.

The physiologic changes associated with normovolemic hemodilution are of current interest, particularly in patients with coronary artery or cerebral vascular disease. Blood viscosity remains good and organ blood flow is maintained if hypotension is avoided. The ability to compensate for low hematocrit by increases in cardiac output and coronary blood flow may be of importance. Experimental evidence in the dog suggests that this compensation for acute changes in hematocrit can persist for several hours, but the presence of severe coronary artery stenosis causes decompensation and regional left ventricular dysfunction.[8,9]

Intraoperative Blood Salvage

Collecting blood intraoperatively entails salvaging blood shed by the patient in the operating room, washing it, and then reinfusing it into the patient. Washing removes debris, anticoagulant, and free hemoglobin. Initially, blood is collected in the reservoir of the Cell Saver,® then pumped into a centrifuge bowl. As the blood spins, supernatant waste, free hemoglobin, anticoagulant, fat, and bone marrow elements are washed off. Continued washing and spinning can increase the hematocrit to 50% to 60%. After washing, the blood is pumped into a transfusion bag and then administered to the patient.

To determine the efficacy of intraoperative cell salvage, we conducted an 18-month survey of 1800 patients undergoing a variety of orthopedic procedures at our institution. Eighty-three percent of patients had blood returned during surgery.[10]

Postoperative Blood Salvage Devices

Blood that is lost into wound drainage devices can be reinfused into the patient. At our institution, we collect blood with a 265-micron filter and reinfuse it through a 40-micron filter (Davol®). The postoperative reinfusion device contains blood that is low in platelets, has elevated fibrin degradation products, low fibrinogen, elevated prothrombin time (PT), partial thromboplastin time (PTT), and some free hemoglobin. The hematocrit of the reinfused blood is slightly lower than systemic levels. Potential risks of the postoperative reinfusion device include renal insufficiency due to hemolyzed cells, dilutional coagulopathy, disseminated intravascular coagulation, complement activation, adult respiratory distress syndrome, and reinfusion of anticoagulants. One report on washed versus unwashed reinfusion of postoperative wound drainage indicates that patients who received unwashed blood had more complications than those who received washed blood.[11] However, analysis of the data demonstrate that two of the patients who received unwashed blood had immediate hypotension, which could result from the infusion of anticoagulant. One patient had an unexplained hyperthermic episode postinfusion, and one patient had hypotension unrelated to blood reinfusion 5 hours postoperatively.

Justification for washing blood prior to reinfusion is not supported by data collected from our institution. We followed up over 1000 patients who received postoperative Davol® infusions, and there were no reported complications.

Avoiding Homologous Blood Transfusion

Results concerning homologous blood-transfusion requirements for patients who have undergone specific procedures show that the need for such transfusions can be greatly reduced. For example, Woolson described 154 primary hip-replacement patients, of whom 92% did not require homologous blood because of the combined use of predeposit blood, Cell Saver, and postoperative salvage.[12] On average, 408 mL of blood was salvaged and reinfused with no complications.

In a 1987 study of patients at our institution, 2 units of predonated blood by itself helped patients avoid homologous transfusions in 75% of cases.[13] In 1990, a combination of 2 predonated units, Cell Saver, and Davol helped avoid homologous blood requirements in 96% of patients. In this study, 233 patients were divided into predonators and nonpredonators; recipients and nonrecipients of Cell Saver; and patients who were reinfused postoperatively and those who were not. Of patients who did not predonate, homologous transfusion was avoided in only 43%, with or without Cell Saver or Davol reinfusion. On the other hand, 85% of patients who predonated 2 units and had Cell Saver use did not require homologous transfusions. These data point up the importance of predonation in hip surgery.

A study of spine surgery by Mann and colleagues showed that with a combination of predeposit and Cell Saver, over 90% of single-stage procedures did not require homologous blood.[14]

In a review at our institution of 24 cases of combined anterior and posterior spinal fusions, 2 of 24 patients received homologous blood. The average blood loss was 1,650 mL the average Cell Saver reinfused was 480 mL, and in 18 patients for whom data were available for Davol reinfusion, reinfusion averaged 430 mL. The admission hematocrit was 35.3%; discharge hematocrit was 30.5%. Two patients received homologous blood; one received 1 unit of blood during the procedure, but when the hematocrit was 21%, the patient did not get a second unit. Three patients received donor-directed blood (personal communication).

Acceptable Hematocrit Levels

In the past, patients were routinely transfused for hematocrit levels of 30%. This no longer appears necessary, as many studies have demonstrated that healthy patients can tolerate levels lower than 30% without complications.[15,16]

When assessing a patient's ability to tolerate low hemoglobin levels, it is important to ensure that oxygen delivery to the tissues is not compromised. Cardiac output and the oxygen content of the arterial blood are two factors that influence this:

$$DO_2 = CaO_2 \times Qt$$

where:
DO_2 = oxygen delivery
CaO_2 = arterial oxygen content
Qt = cardiac output

The oxygen content is determined by the hemoglobin concentration and the percentage of that hemoglobin that is saturated with oxygen ($SO_2\%$):

$$CaO_2 = (Hb \times 1.34) \times SO_2\% + (0.0031 \times PaO_2)$$

These equations show that cardiac output may be an important factor in a patient's tolerance of acute anemia.

The decision to transfuse should be based on the patient's physiologic status, actual and anticipated blood loss, ability to compensate for anemia, and oxygen requirements.[17]

References

1. Fernandez MC, Gottlieb M, Menitove JE. Blood transfusion and postoperative infection in orthopedic patients. *Transfusion* 1992;32(4):318-322.

2. Zauder HL. Preoperative hemoglobin requirements. In: Spiess BD, ed. *Hemorrhagic Disorders*. Anesthesiology Clinics of North America. Philadelphia, Pa: WB Saunders; 1990;8:471.

3. McVay PA, Andrews A, Hoag MS, et al. Moderate and severe reactions during autologous blood donations are no more frequent than during homologous blood donations. *Vox Sang* 1990;59(2):70-72.

4. Toy P. Autologous Transfusion. In: Spiess BD, ed. *Hemorrhagic Disorders*. Anesthesiology Clinics of North America. Philadelphia, Pa: WB Saunders; 1990;8:533.

5. MacEwen GD, Bennett E, Guille JT. Autologous blood transfusions in children and young adults with low body weight undergoing spinal surgery. *J Pediatr Orthop* 1990;10(6):750-753.

6. Goodnough LT, Rudnick S, Price TH, et al. Increased preoperative collection of autologous blood with recombinant human erythropoietin therapy. *N Engl J Med* 1989;321(17):1163-1168.

7. Lorentz A, Jendrissek A, Eckardt KU, Schipplick M, Osswald PM, Kurtz A. Serial immunoreactive erythropoietin levels in autologous blood donors. *Transfusion* 1991;31:650-654.

8. Spahn DR, Smith LR, McRae RL, Leone BJ. Effects of acute isovolemic hemodilution and anesthesia on regional function in left ventricular myocardium with compromised coronary blood flow. *Acta Anaesthesiol Scand* 1992;36:628-636.

9. Bowens C, Spahn D, Frasco P, Smith LR, McRae RL, Leone BJ. Hemodilution induces stable changes in global cardiovascular and regional myocardial function. *Anesth Analg* 1993;76:1027-1032.

10. Bernstein D, Rosenberg AD, Blackshear C. Intraoperative cell salvage in orthopedic surgery. *Anesth Analg* 1994;78:S37.

11. Clements DH, Sculco TP, Burke SW, Mayer K, Levine D. Salvage and reinfusion of postoperative sanguineous wound drainage. *J Bone Joint Surg* 1992;74A:646-651.

12. Woolson ST, Marsh JS, Tanner J. Transfusion of previously deposited autologous blood for patients undergoing hip replacement surgery. *J Bone Joint Surg* 1987;69A:325-328.

13. Rosenberg AD, Bernstein DB, Ramanathan S. What is the best method to avoid homologous transfusion? *Anesthesiology* 1990;73:A1016.

14. Mann DC, Wilham MR, Brower EM, Nash C Jr. Decreasing homologous blood transfusion in spinal surgery by use of the cell saver and predeposited blood. *Spine* 1989;14(12):1296-1300.

15. Stehling L. Perioperative mortality in anemic patients. *Transfusion* 1989;29:37S.

16. Nelson AH, Fleisher LA, Rosenbaum SH. Relationship between postoperative anemia and cardiac morbidity in high-risk vascular patients in the intensive care unit. *Crit Care Med* 1993;21(6):860-866.

17. Stehling L, Simon TL. The red blood cell transfusion trigger. physiology and clinical studies. *Arch Pathol Lab Med* 1994;118(4):429-434.

Effects of Joint Replacement
on the Coagulation System

Ola E. Dahl, MD

Hip replacement surgery with acrylic cement for prosthesis fixation is associated with significant intraoperative and postoperative morbidity and mortality. The incidence of sudden death from intraoperative cardiorespiratory dysfunction in published studies ranges from 0.02% to 11% and mortality due to pulmonary embolism ranges from 2% to 3%.[1-4] Complex orthopedic surgery is highly traumatic and may be complicated by substantial intraoperative blood loss and serious postoperative thromboembolic events.

Postoperative deep-vein thrombosis (DVT) occurs in up to 60% of patients given inadequate thromboprophylaxis and is even higher when no thromboprophylaxis is given.[5-7] At Ulleval University Hospital (Oslo), we have estimated a blood loss on average of 1600 mL in over 300 patients who had hip-replacement surgery. Most of these patients had cement-anchored prostheses (80%). Bleeding was approximately 500 to 1000 mL more in patients in whom prosthesis were implanted without cement, probably because the bone cavity had not been plugged with cement. After revision arthroplasty, we have noted even higher blood loss, which in single patients may reach 5 to 6 liters (unpublished data).

Vascular hemostasis requires a fine balance between the coagulation and fibrinolytic systems. Any imbalance may lead to abnormal bleeding or thrombosis formation. Mechanical bone traumatization, including impaction of bone cement into the femoral cavity, will cause the release of bone marrow content into venous blood. This bone marrow contains procoagulant cells and debris that will lead to local activation of the coagulation cascade in the blood draining the operation field.

Systemic Activation of Coagulation

In patients undergoing total hip replacement surgery, frequent blood samples were obtained from the pulmonary artery (mixed venous blood = MVB) and from the radial artery (arterial blood = AB) and markers of activation of the coagulation cascade were analyzed.[8] The protocol for blood sampling is shown in Table 1. Only small decreases were found in the activity of the intrinsic kallikrein-kinin contact system and in the complement system. However, during bone preparation, a marked fall in factor VII (Fig 1) and a substantial increase in fibrinopeptide A (FPA [Fig 2]) occurred in the arterial blood compared with much smaller changes in the blood sampled from the pulmonary artery. Maximal levels of FPA were reached at the time of the acetabular implantation and thereafter decreased to preoperative levels 1 hour after surgery. The significantly higher levels of FPA in arterial blood leaving the lungs indicate a substantial capacity of the lung vascular system for thrombin generation and fibrin formation when blood-borne procoagulant debris from traumatized bone tissue passes through the lung capillaries. This finding has been confirmed by the measurement of thrombin-antithrombin III (TAT) complexes (Fig 3) and prothrombin activation fragments 1 + 2 (F1+2[Fig 4])[9,10]. Thus, hypercoagulable blood is squeezed out of the lungs into the peripheral circulation and may favor thrombosis formation in central and peripheral microcapillaries and in larger collecting veins.

Table 1. Blood Sampling Times in Patients Undergoing Total Hip-Replacement Surgery	
Sample Number	Surgical Procedure
1	After induction of epidural analgesia
2	After femoral osteotomy
3	After bone preparation
4	Acetabular implantation
5	10 min later
6	Femoral implantation
7	10 min later
8	1 h after surgery
9	Postop day 1
10	Postop day 3
11	Postop day 6

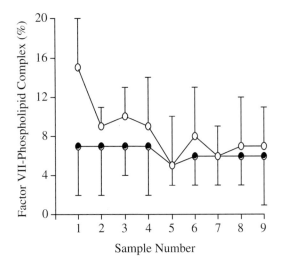

Fig 1. Intraoperative values of factor VII-phospholipid complex in mixed venous blood (MVB)• – • and arterial blood (AB) o – o . Mean ± SEM Sampling: Table 1.
Dahl OE, Molnar I, Vinje A, et al. Studies on coagulation, fibrinolysis, kallikrein-kinin and complement activation in systemic and pulmonary circulation during hip arthroplasty with acrylic cement. *Thromb Res* 1988;50(6):875-84.

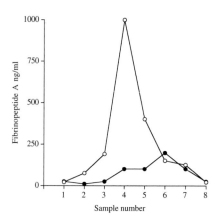

Fig 2. Intraoperative values of fibrinopeptide A in mixed venous blood (MVB) • – •
and arterial blood (AB) o – o blood. Sampling: Table 1. Redrawn from: Dahl OE,
Molnar I, Vinje A, et al. Studies on coagulation, fibrinolysis, kallikrein-kinin and
complement activation in systemic and pulmonary circulation during hip arthroplasty
with acrylic cement. *Thromb Res* 1988;50(6):875-84.

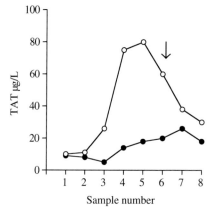

Fig 3. Thrombin-antithrombin III (TAT) complexes appeared early during
preparation of bone in significantly higher amounts in arterial blood (AB) o – o than
in mixed venous blood (MVB) • – • , indicating generation of thrombin during
passage of blood through the lungs. (down arrow) : impaction of cement and
prosthesis into the femoral shaft. Sampling: Table 1 Redrawn from: Dahl OE,
Johnsen H, Kierulf P, et al. Intrapulmonary thrombin generation and its relation to
monomethylmethacrylate plasma levels during hip arthroplasty. *Acta Anaesthesiol
Scand* 1992;36(4):331-5.

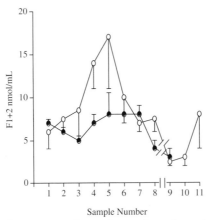

Fig 4. Intraoperative and postoperative values of prothrombin fragments (F1+2) in mixed venous blood (MVB) ●–● and arterial blood (AB) o – o. Mean ± SEM Sampling: Table 1. Redrawn from: Dahl OE, Pedersen T, Kierulf P, et al. Sequential intrapulmonary and systemic activation of coagulation and fibrinolysis during and after total hip replacement surgery. *Thromb Res* 1993;70(6):451-8.

Impaired Fibrinolysis

The massive intraoperative activation of coagulation seen in the patients undergoing hip replacement surgery was followed by activation of fibrinolysis (Fig 5).[10] Tissue plasminogen activator (t-PA) antigen was significantly elevated by the end of the surgery. This was counteracted by an antifibrinolytic response and an increase in plasminogen activator inhibitor type 1 activity (PAI-1) on the first postoperative day (Fig 6). Fibrinolytic shutdown occurred between the first and the third postoperative day as evidenced by a fall in t-PA (Fig 5) and also in the fibrin split products (D-dimers) that had been rising throughout surgery and the immediate postoperative period.

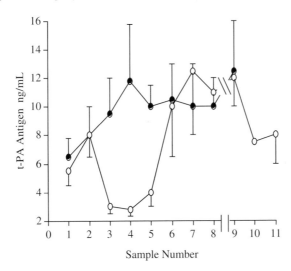

Fig 5. Intraoperative and postoperative values of tissue plasminogen activator (t-PA) antigen in mixed venous blood (MVB) ● – ● and arterial blood (AB) o – o. Mean ± SEM Sampling: Table 1. Redrawn from: Dahl OE, Pedersen T, Kierulf P, et al. Sequential intrapulmonary and systemic activation of coagulation and fibrinolysis during and after total hip replacement surgery. *Thromb Res* 1993;70(6):451-8.

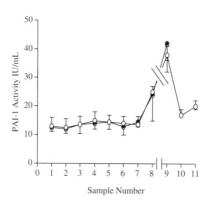

Sample Number

Fig 6. Intraoperative and postoperative values of plasminogen activator inhibitor type 1 (PAI-1) activity in mixed venous blood (MVB) • – • and arterial blood (AB) o – o . Mean ± SEM Sampling: Table 1. Redrawn from: Dahl OE, Pedersen T, Kierulf P, et al. Sequential intrapulmonary and systemic activation of coagulation and fibrinolysis during and after total hip replacement surgery. *Thromb Res* 1993;70(6):451-8.

The PAI-1 increase on postoperative day 1 was paralleled by an increase in the acute-phase cytokine, interleukin-6 (IL-6), which can stimulate tissue factor expression on vascular endothelial cells.[10,11] This may have contributed to a second wave of coagulation activity that was seen at the end of the first postoperative week and resulted in a further rise in F1+2 activity (See Fig 4).

These data would suggest an imbalance between activation of the coagulation and fibrinolytic systems, with a bias towards a procoagulant state in these patients both during surgery and at the end of the first postoperative week.

Prolonged Activation of Coagulation
We followed up more than 300 hip-replacement surgical patients after hospital discharge to study the frequency of DVT and PE up until 5 weeks after surgery and to evaluate effects of prolonged thromboprophylaxis.[12] As part of this study, a secondary substudy investigated any prolonged effects of the surgery on hemostasis and fibrinolysis in patients with and without prolonged thromboprophylaxis with dalteparin. Measurements of markers of coagulation and fibrinolysis showed that a prolonged hypercoagulable state existed for at least 5 weeks in patients without continuing prophylaxis compared to patients with thromboprophylaxis for only one week.[13] Figures 7 and 8 summarize the effects in patients with and without prolonged prophylaxis and show elevated levels of TAT and D -dimers, indicating continual activation of the coagulation cascade. The t-PA antigen levels were low, indicating impaired fibrinolysis (Fig 9). During this period (day 7 to day 35), the overall incidence of DVT frequency from 16% to 25%.

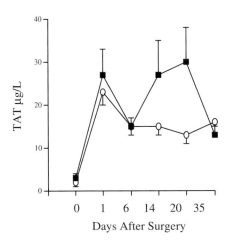

Fig 7. Plasma thrombin-antithrombin III (TAT) complexes (mean ± SEM) in hip-replacement surgery patients without prophylaxis (filled squares, n = 5) and with prophylaxis (open circles, n= 7) until 35 days after surgery. From: Dahl O, Aspelin T, Arnesen H, et al. Increased activation of coagulation and formation of deep vein thrombosis following hip replacement surgery. *Thromb Res*. 1995;80:299-306.

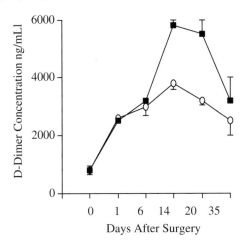

Fig 8. Plasma D-dimer levels (mean ± SEM) in hip-replacement surgery patients without prophylaxis (filled squares, n = 5) and with prophylaxis (open circles, n= 7) until 35 days after surgery. Redrawn from: Dahl OE, Westvik AB, Kierulf P, Lyberg T. Effect of monomethylmethacrylate on procoagulant activities of human monocytes and umbilical vein endothelial cells in vitro. *Thromb Res* 1995;80:299-306.

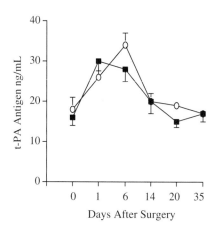

Fig 9. Plasma tissue plasminogen activator (t-PA) antigen levels (mean ± SEM) in hip-replacement surgery patients without prophylaxis (filled squares, n = 5) and with prophylaxis (open circles, n= 7) until 35 days after surgery. *Thromb Res* 1995;80:299-306.

Role of Bone Cement in Activating Coagulation

Bone cement may contribute to activation of coagulation (1) mechanically, by causing release of procoagulant bone marrow debris into venous blood when the cement is pressed into the bone cavity and when the prosthesis is pressed into the impacted cement; and (2) chemically, because methylmethacrylate (MMA) monomer, a main component of bone cement, is clearly cytotoxic in high concentrations[14] and may cause endothelial cell disruption and detachment in veins close to cemented areas, resulting in exposure of subendothelial procoagulants. This may possibly form nidi for thrombosis formation.

Animal Studies

To investigate in more detail what happens in venous blood at the site of surgery, hip-replacement operations were performed on domestic pigs.[15] Sixteen animals were studied; eight had prosthetic fixation with acrylic cement and eight had implantation without cement. Blood samples were obtained from femoral veins in both the operated and nonoperated limbs at various time points until 90 minutes after surgery. Markers of activation of the coagulation and fibrinolytic systems were analyzed. A marked rise in TAT, ie, activation of coagulation, appeared in femoral vein blood on the operated side compared with the nonoperated side during bone preparation. This was followed by a short, intense burst of fibrinolytic activity (rise in t-PA), which was counteracted by an antifibrinolytic process (rise in PAI-1) after implantation of the femoral prosthesis. Results in the noncemented group were similar, with significantly higher levels on the operated side compared with the nonoperated side. However, overall activation of coagulation and the fibrinolytic responses were attenuated in animals not exposed to acrylic cement.

Electron microscopic examination of the femoral veins from these animals showed signs of DVT, with fibrin deposits and platelet aggregates in 62% of animals with cemented prostheses compared with 25% of animals in whom cement was not used. All these histologic findings were in femoral veins taken from the operated side of the animals. On the unoperated side, regular endothelial lining with only spots of fibrin deposits were seen in both groups.

In vitro Studies

An in vitro study has demonstrated that MMA alone or in combination with thrombin has effects on monocytes to modulate their procoagulant activity.[16] Moderate doses of MMA alone had a slight tissue factor-expressing effect on monocytes (Fig 10 A). Small doses of MMA in combination with fixed doses of thrombin markedly potentiated the tissue factor expression (Fig 10 A,B). This up-regulation of tissue factor expression on monocytes may contribute to activation of coagulation by binding to factor VII and thereby initiating the extrinsic coagulation system. Methylmethacrylate monomer can also destroy other cells such as leukocytes and cause release of intracellular proteolytic enzymes, which further contribute to vascular destruction and exposure of subendothelial procoagulant constituents.[14]

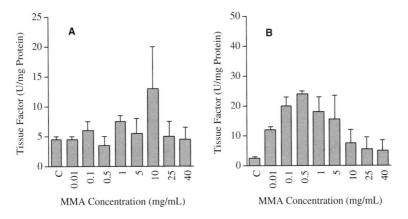

Fig 10. Tissue factor expression of monocytes exposed to different concentrations of methylmethacrylate (MMA). A, MMA stimulation alone B, MMA co-stimulated with thrombin (10 U/mL); C = unstimulated control cells. Mean ± SEM. *Thromb Res* 1994;74:377-387.

SUMMARY

The bone traumatization that occurs as a result of hip-replacement surgery causes bleeding; impaction of bone cement plugs the bone cavity and reduces blood loss but also increases the local and systemic activation of coagulation that occurs both during and after surgery. Thus, patients undergoing this type of surgery appear to have an unbalanced activation of coagulation and fibrinolysis, with an overload of procoagulant activity both during and after surgery, although marked perioperative bleeding may still occur.

References

1.   Charnley J. Risks of total hip replacement. *Br Med J* 1975;4:101. Letter.

2. Duncan JA. Intra-operative collapse or death related to the use of acrylic cement in hip surgery. *Anaesthesia* 1989;44:149-153. Comments.

3. Dahl OE, Molnar I, Ro JS, Vinje A. Global tests on coagulation and fibrinolysis in systemic and pulmonary circulation accompanying hip arthroplasty with acrylic cement. *Thromb Res* 1988;50:865-873.

4. Bergqvist D. *Postoperative Thromboembolism. Frequency, Etiology, Prophylaxis.* New York: Springer-Verlag; 1983.

5. Nillius A, Nylander G. Deep vein thrombosis after total hip replacement: a clinical and phlebographic study. *Br J Surg* 1979;66:324-326.

6. Stamatakis JD, Kakkar VV, Sagar S, Lawrence D, Nairn D, Bentley PG. Femoral vein thrombosis and total hip replacement. *Br Med J* 1977;2:223-225.

7. Kalodiki E, Nicolaides A, Al-Kutoubi A, Birch R, Harris N. LMWH and LMWH plus graduated elastic compression for DVT prophylaxis in total hip replacement. *Thromb Haemost* 1993;69:619.

8. Dahl OE, Molnar I, Vinje A, et al. Studies on coagulation, fibrinolysis, kallikrein-kinin and complement activation in systemic and pulmonary circulation during hip arthroplasty with acrylic cement. *Thromb Res* 1988;50:875-884.

9. Dahl OE, Johnsen H, Kierulf P, et al. Intrapulmonary thrombin generation and its relation to monomethylmethacrylate plasma levels during hip arthroplasty. *Acta Anaesthesiol Scand* 1992;36:331-335.

10. Dahl OE, Pedersen T, Kierulf P, et al. Sequential intrapulmonary and systemic activation of coagulation and fibrinolysis during and after total hip replacement surgery. *Thromb Res* 1993;70:451-458.

11. Salgado A, Boveda JL, Monasterio J, et al. Inflammatory mediators and their influence on haemostasis. *Haemostasis* 1994;24:132-138.

12. Dahl O, Andreassen G, Muller C, et al. Prolonged thromboprophylaxis following hip replacement surgerey – Results of a double-blind, prospective, randomized, placebo-controlled study with dalteparin (Fragmin R). *Lancet* 1996 (Submitted).

13. Dahl O, Aspelin T, Arnesen H, et al. Increased activation of coagulation and formation of deep vein thrombosis following hip replacement surgery. *Thromb Res* 1995:80:299-306.

14. Dahl OE, Garvik LJ, Lyberg T. Toxic effects of methylmethacrylate monomer on leukocytes and endothelial cells in vitro. *Acta Orthop Scand* 1994;65:147-153.

15. Dahl OE, Aspelin T, Lyberg T. The role of bone traumatization in the initiation of proximal deep vein thrombosis during hip replacement surgery in pigs. *Blood Coag Fibrinol* 1995;6:709-717.

16. Dahl OE, Westvik AB, Kierulf P, Lyberg T. Effect of monomethylmethacrylate on procoagulant activities of human monocytes and umbilical vein endothelial cells in vitro. *Thromb Res* 1994;74:377-387.

Perioperative Bleeding in Spinal Surgery: Identification and Management

Robert Mervyn Letts MD, FRCSC

Blood loss during surgery and in the postoperative phase has always been of great concern to surgeons. Spinal surgery, a delicate and technically demanding procedure, requires the surgeon to have a clear view of the spinal elements to perform the technical maneuver necessary to correct the problem at hand. Significant hemorrhage obscures the field, making it extremely difficult to perform surgery in the safest possible manner. The emergence of the human immuno-deficiency virus (HIV) as well as the various strains of hepatitis virus has intensified the concern of surgeons regarding blood loss during surgical procedures. This is especially true of spinal surgeons, who deal with large wounds with the potential for significant bleeding. Blood salvage techniques have greatly reduced the need for homologous blood transfusions, but it is the surgeon's responsibility to keep blood loss to a minimum and to keep transfusion requirements to the least number of units possible. The AIDS epidemic has prompted a rethinking of the level of circulating hemoglobin necessary for a safe existence and for good wound healing.[1] A decade ago, we were reluctant to let the hemoglobin fall below 10 g and the hematocrit below 30 (the old 10/30 rule).

We now almost routinely never transfuse above 8 g or a 25% hematocrit. Technology for cell savers has improved immensely; in addition, almost all blood banks can now collect at least 3 units due to better preservatives in almost all patients seen preoperatively. New drugs and pharmaceuticals that decrease bleeding or increase erythropoiesis hold great promise in controlling surgical blood loss and minimizing the requirements for transfusion. Recombinant erythropoietic hormone, ie erythropoietin, has particular promise in this regard.[2] Thus, there are a number of techniques and new discoveries now available to surgeons to assist in avoiding transfusions and minimizing blood loss in spinal surgery.

Preoperative Identification of Potential Bleeding

Many bleeding problems can be recognized and corrected prior to spinal surgery. This includes taking a good personal and family history of previous bleeding disorders. Bleeding problems encountered during dental work, for example, is often very beneficial in spotting mild degrees of von Willebrand's disease that can be effectively treated with desmopressin (DDAVP) prior to surgery. A history of the pharmaceuticals and drugs being taken is absolutely essential. Many drugs (eg, salicylates, nonsteroidal anti-inflammatories, or anticoagulants) may increase bleeding (Table 1), and many of them need only be stopped prior to surgery to eliminate the bleeding risk. By identifying preoperative causes of potential surgical bleeding, appropriate management to decrease hemorrhage during the procedure and eliminate a major cause of blood loss can be undertaken.

Table 1. Drugs That May Increase Bleeding	
• Anticoagulants (heparin, warfarin)	• Radiographic contrast agents
• Antibiotics	• Volume expanders
• Antithrombotics (dipyridamole)	• Volatile anesthetics
• Nonsteroidal anti-inflammatory drugs	• Other drugs (antihistamines)
• Cardioactive and vaso\active drugs	

PREOPERATIVE DIAGNOSIS

It is essential that other associated medical conditions that may predispose to bleeding be diagnosed accurately prior to surgery. For example, scoliosis itself is felt to have an inherent platelet abnormality in as high as 50% of patients, with some 25% of scoliosis patients possibly having collagen abnormalities that predispose to bleeding.[3] It is well recognized that children with neuromuscular spinal abnormalities frequently bleed more profusely than normal; for example, muscular dystrophy, spina bifida, spinal muscular atrophy or collagen disorders such as Ehlers-Danlos syndrome or Marfan's syndrome. Knowing the associated diagnosis sensitizes the health-care team to the possibility of excessive bleeding and steps can be taken to counteract the hemorrhage.[4]

PREOPERATIVE PREPARATION

Preoperative preparation for major spinal surgery is important to minimize bleeding. There are a myriad of spinal implants on the market today, and spinal surgeons have to be familiar with a number of them, especially those used to solve the particular problem at hand. It is therefore important that if a procedure utilizing a new implant is to be used, the whole health-care team should be made familiar with the equipment and its application. This will assist in decreasing the operative time and, hence, reduce the risk time for bleeding. The operative team is one of the most important factors in minimizing blood loss, since the more efficient the team, the less the time required for surgery and the more efficient the hemostasis. In this regard, one can anticipate the magnitude of intraoperative bleeding by the number of levels to be fused, the age of the patient, the presence of obesity, or how much bone graft will be required. The younger patient, ie, the child under 12 years of age, usually has a very well-developed periosteum and by decorticating this subperiosteally, bleeding is often lessened. In older teenagers and adults, there is very little periosteum and the bleeding is therefore more profuse. There is a direct correlation between the amount of bleeding and the number of levels being fused in spine surgery. This also necessitates greater amounts of bone graft requiring more dissection of the iliac crest. Thus preoperative decisions such as the use of bone bank bone or having an extra assistant for longer fusions or ensuring a cell saver is in the operating room will all bear on reducing blood loss.

INTRAOPERATIVE BLEEDING
Increased Venous Compression

Batson[5] in 1940 first recognized that the increased incidence of metastasis in the lumbar spine was secondary to a complex venous system connecting abdominal and pelvic veins to the vertebral venous system. He demonstrated that increased compression on abdominal contents could force blood containing malignant cells into the spinal venous system. These veins, now commonly referred to as Batson's veins are of major concern to spinal surgeons. If there is increased abdominal pressure, these veins are distended and prone to bleed excessively. To minimize intra-abdominal pressure, spinal surgeons have used special spinal supports for a number of years. These include the Relton-Hall[6] frame or the Hastings[7] frame, which allows the abdominal contents to fall forward and not rest on the inferior vena cava, creating a back flow through Batson's veins and into the area of spine that is being operated upon. This is a very effective way of physically reducing bleeding.[8]

Skin and Small-Vessel Bleeding

The first bleeding encountered in any surgery is from the small vessels that are cut in exposing the spine. An epinephrine solution can minimize this to some extent. A 1/500,000 epinephrine solution injected into the wound site prior to the incision helps to reduce this type of bleeding. Certain medical abnormalities predispose to bleeding at this stage as well, notably neuromuscular abnormalities or paraplegia where the muscular layer of the arterioles is also hypotonic, resulting in an inability for the vessel to close during the vascular phase of bleeding. Cutting cautery or laser scalpels help to reduce this type of troublesome oozing.

Platelet Abnormalities

Patients with platelet abnormalities that have been identified preoperatively can be treated both preoperatively and intraoperatively with appropriate counteragents. For example, a patient with von Willebrand's syndrome can be administered DDAVP both preoperatively and intraoperatively to control the platelet abnormality.[9,10] There are some patients with no identified abnormality who may experience excessive initial bleeding despite a normal bleeding screen. This is not uncommonly observed in patients with neuromuscular abnormalities and in the occasional child undergoing surgery for idiopathic scoliosis. In such instances, DDAVP may assist in reducing this troublesome bleeding, which may be due to an unrecognized platelet abnormality. As well, the technique of immediately applying self-retaining retractors to the wound will greatly assist in stopping skin bleeding and bleeding in the subcutaneous tissue simply by their traction effect. This, of course, needs to be supplemented with meticulous cautery hemostasis of larger vessel bleeding.

Desmopressin: An Adjunct to Hemostasis?

The antidiuretic hormone vasopressin, the peptide produced by the posterior pituitary, was initially used in the treatment of diabetes insipidus. Because of its extremely short half-life and very significant vasoconstrictive activity, scientists in the former Czechoslovakia developed the vasopressin analog 1-deamino-8-D-arginine vasopressin (DDAVP), or desmopressin, in 1963. This drug is now the preferred medication for diabetes insipidus due to its very potent antidiuretic properties, lack of vasoconstrictive effects, and a much greater half-life than any antidiuretic hormone.[11]

Dosage. Desmopressin is administered at a dosage of 10 $\mu g/m^2$ per square meter of body surface area, with a maximum dosage of 20 μg. It is diluted to a final concentration of 0.5 $\mu g/mL$ in physiologic saline and infused intravenously over a 20-minute period by the anesthetist at the start of surgery.

Hemostatic Properties. It has been demonstrated in two laboratories that DDAVP enhances the circulating levels of factor VIII, von Willebrand factor, and plasminogen activator for at least 6 hours postadministration. Accompanying the increase in these parameters is a decrease in partial thromboplastin and bleeding times and increased fibrinolysis.[11,12] These changes have been shown to occur in normal individuals, as well as in those with bleeding disorders. Thus, DDAVP is the drug of choice in the treatment of von Willebrand's disease or bleeding secondary to excessive salicylate ingestion. It should be emphasized that although few studies have addressed the effects of DDAVP specifically in children, clinical use of desmopressin has been largely in the pediatric population. The exact mechanism of DDAVP action on other aspects of the blood coagulation mechanism is unknown. An increase in platelet aggregation is accompanied by a fall in the platelet count and there may be a direct effect of DDAVP on the blood vessel wall cell membranes, perhaps mediated by the V2 vasopressin receptor.[10] Some investigators have shown increased platelet adhesion and endothelial cell spreading at sites of vascular injury after DDAVP therapy.[11]

Influence of DDAVP on Surgical Blood Loss

Major surgical procedures such as cardiac and orthopedic surgery accompanied by large blood loss may have continued bleeding secondary to thrombocytopenia, platelet defects, decreases in concentration of clotting factors and fibrinolysis. The use of DDAVP in cardiac surgery has now been studied in several centers.[10-12] Czer et al[13] in well-controlled double-blind studies concluded that this agent reduced blood loss in patients undergoing complex cardiac operations. More recently, Hedderich and coworkers[14] and Rocha et al[15] could not demonstrate significant differences in intraoperative blood loss in routine coronary artery bypass surgery or valvular and congenital heart surgery. Kobrinsky and associates[10] in a study of the effects of DDAVP on the blood loss in patients undergoing major spinal surgery found significant reduction in the blood loss in patients with neuromuscular scoliosis, with less reduction in patients with idiopathic scoliosis who underwent spinal fusion. It is interesting that through the release of prostacyclin, DDAVP should induce vasodilatation rather than vasoconstriction and hence one might expect a worsening of the bleeding in those patients with neuromuscular disease and poorer vascular tone! How DDAVP decreases operative blood loss in this group of patients is not clear, but through the augmentation of hemostasis, it can obviously overcome a bleeding tendency induced by poor vascular tone. It would appear that DDAVP has less effect on patients with normal hematologic and vascular parameters such as is usually seen in most patients with idiopathic scoliosis or those undergoing "routine" coronary bypass or valvular cardiac surgery. There does, however, seem to be a very beneficial effect of DDAVP in patients undergoing surgery with known abnormalities in platelets or small vessels. Its exact role in preventing blood loss in major surgical procedures is still not clear, but there is no question that some patients respond to it with marked decrease in blood loss. Further studies are needed to ascertain the most appropriate class of patient to whom DDAVP should be administered preoperatively. The reduction of even one unit of blood requirement ie 300 to 500 cc of blood loss, may allow such patients to have this major procedure performed using only their predonated blood, thus decreasing the risk of blood-borne diseases such as hepatitis or AIDS. In patients undergoing instrumentation and spinal fusion, these groups appear to be the neuromuscularly compromised group, in particular, cerebral palsy and spina bifida patients. Indeed platelet disorders have been identified by Yarom and coworkers[16] in both scoliosis and muscular dystrophy, which may explain the response to DDAVP seen in some of these patients.

Experience of the Surgeon and Surgical Team

The experience and skill of the surgeon, backed by a knowledgeable and supportive team can greatly decrease the length of time of the surgery and, consequently, the amount of bleeding encountered. Familiarity with the equipment, technique, and routine involved in a surgical procedure decreases the multiple small delays that can occur when the surgical team is not sufficiently experienced with the operation being performed. These delays significantly prolong the operative procedure and the bleeding occasioned by prolonged surgery. Dedicated personnel, appropriate surgical instruments, a choice of implants, and easy access to a bone bank are essential elements of a smooth, efficient operating team that will ensure the procedure is accomplished safely and effectively with minimal surgical time.

Sequence of the Surgical Procedure

Increased bleeding is often encountered if the sequence of the surgical procedure is not efficient. For example, in spinal fusion the decortication should be deferred until the end of the procedure to minimize the time of excessive bone bleeding. It is good technique to move from one part of the wound to another. When bleeding is encountered that can not quickly be controlled, that part of the wound should be packed and attention directed to another part of the wound. The bone graft site can initially be exposed, packed to control oozing, and the graft taken only towards the end of the procedure, again to minimize the bleeding from decorticated bone surfaces. Occasionally, profuse bleeding is encountered from a bone artery or a nutrient vessel; and this can usually be controlled with bone wax or direct cautery or both.[17]

Hemostatic Equipment

Cutting lasers are being improved to the point that their use greatly minimizes bleeding. This can also be accomplished with cutting cautery techniques, which are especially useful in situations that are known to produce excessive bleeding, eg, in the hemophiliac patient, when the vascular phase of bleeding is compromised, or when cutting through muscle.

The Bone Graft

Because autologous bone graft is more efficient in promoting union, this type of graft is preferred by most surgeons and is usually harvested from the iliac crest. The iliac crest can be a significant source of bleeding and certainly adds to the overall bleeding encountered in spinal surgery. It is essential that the anatomy of this area, as well as the anatomy of the entire spine, be intimately known by the surgeon to avoid the major adjacent large vessels. The gluteal vessels in the region of the iliac crest are vessels that can bleed profusely. The correct technique of taking the graft is essential to avoid excessive bleeding in the region of the ilium. Thus, subperiosteal dissection and staying out of the muscle mass will greatly minimize bleeding in this area. Misadventures such as "plunging" may result in major gluteal vessel injury. By exposing the ilium first and packing with a large Raytex, troublesome bleeding can be controlled and stopped prior to the taking of the actual graft at a later stage in the procedure. Bleeding from the raw graft surface is usually quite controllable with gel foam.

Decortication Bleeding

Decortication of the spine in preparation for spinal fusion should be deferred until close to the end of the procedure. This decreases the time of potential bleeding from the raw bone surface. Bleeding that is profuse or cannot be controlled can be managed with thrombin-soaked gel foam or, occasionally, bone wax, although this may inhibit fusion when used excessively.

Laminectomy Bleeding

Bleeding encountered during laminectomies is usually venous but can be significant and troublesome. Thrombin-soaked pledgets introduced into the canal usually control this type of bleeding. Other topical agents such as Avertin, a type of microfibular collagen, can also be used to assist in controlling persistent oozing.[18]

Major Vessel Injury

An intimate knowledge of anatomy by the spinal surgeon as well as the assistants on the team is necessary to avoid major vascular trauma. This seldom occurs in posterior spinal approaches but must be recognized when such injuries do occur. Traversing the anterior longitudinal ligament in disc removal can result in major injury to the aorta or iliac vessels. In such instances, it is of the utmost importance to recognize that this has happened and to turn the patient over and approach the vessel from the front and correct the damage. Large vessels are more prone to injury during anterior approach to the spine but are more readily identified and the hemorrhage more easily dealt with. In most instances, the anterior spinal fusion is associated with less bleeding than posterior spinal fusions.

Anesthesia and Surgical Bleeding

The anesthetist can be the most important assessor of blood loss during spinal surgery. By controlling the blood pressure in a controlled manner during the surgery, hypotension can reduce the amount of bleeding through severed vessels in both bone and soft tissues.[19,20] It is obvious that induced hypotension by an anesthesiologist not skilled in the technique may result in an unfavorable risk:benefit ratio. Induced hypotension to reduce bleeding requires an increased level of patient monitoring and, hence, an anesthetist familiar with this type of surgery. This is especially important if other techniques such as isovolemic hemodilution techniques are to be used, whereby a portion of the patient's blood volume is withdrawn and stored in the immediate presurgical period and reinfused during surgery.[21,22] The exact level at which the mean arterial pressure (MAP) should be maintained during spinal surgery is not clear, but in a recent study Lawhon et al[23] demonstrated that intraoperative bleeding was reduced if the MAP was reduced below 90 mm Hg compared with over 90 mm Hg. They found no extra benefit in lowering the MAP further. Hypotensive anesthesia appears to effect its decrease in blood flow primarily by reducing the left ventricular stroke work index.[24] There has always been concern about hypotensive anesthesia and its effect on spinal cord blood flow and hence predisposing the cord to neurologic injury. It appears, however, that spinal cord blood flow can be autoregulated independently of systemic blood flow under controlled hypotension.[25]

Intraoperative Blood Salvage

The use of a cell saver in spinal surgery has been useful in adults,[26] but not as efficient in children. Unless the loss is in excess of about 1800 mL, the cell saver is not very efficient. For young children, it is not necessary to use the cell saver; for teenagers, it should be reserved for those in whom the blood loss is expected to be in excess of 1800 mL.[27] The use of predeposited autologous blood is the most cost effective and practical method of avoiding homologous blood transfusion during major spinal surgery in children.[28,29]

POSTOPERATIVE BLOOD LOSS

Postoperative blood loss after major posterior spinal fusion averages about 1000 mL. The use of the hemovac to drain spinal wounds is controversial. Having a patient lie on the back for 6 to 8 hours postop tends to tamponade the bleeding, whereas the hemovac may accentuate the bleeding from raw bone surfaces. If a hemovac is to be used, consideration of a cell saver device is recommended.

SUMMARY

Blood loss during spinal surgery has always been of major concern to surgeons. A careful preoperative history and physical examination combined with meticulous surgical technique are essential in minimizing blood loss. The addition of new pharmacologic agents, preoperative blood banking, cell savers, and modern hemostatic agents are all in the armamentarium of the surgical team working to reduce blood loss.

References

1. Welch HG, Meehan KR, Goodnough LT. Prudent strategies for elective red blood cell transfusion. *Ann Intern Med* 1992;116(5):393-402. Comments.

2. Goodnough LT, Rudnick S, Price TH, et al. Increased preoperative collection of autologous blood with recombinant human erythropoietin therapy. *N Engl J Med* 1989;321(17):1163-1168. Comments.

3. Kahmann RD, Donohue JM, Bradford DS, White JG, Rao GH. Platelet function in adolescent idiopathic scoliosis. *Spine* 1992;17(2):145-148.

4. Nelson CL, Nelson RL, Cone J. Blood conservation techniques in orthopaedic surgery. *Instr Course Lect* 1990;39:425-429.

5. Batson OV. The function of the vertebral veins and their role in the spread of metastasis. *Ann Surg* 1940;112:138.

6. Relton JE, Hall JE. An operation frame for spinal fusion: a new apparatus designed to reduce haemorrhage during operation. *J Bone Joint Surg Br* 1967;49(2):327-332.

7. Hastings DE. A simple frame for operations on the lumbar spine. *Can J Surg* 1969;12(2):251-253.

8. Bostman O, Hyrkas J, Hirvensalo E, Kallio E. Blood loss, operating time, and positioning of the patient in lumbar disc surgery. *Spine* 1990;15(5):360-363.

9. Johnson RG, Murphy M, Miller M. Fusions and transfusions: an analysis of blood loss and autologous replacement during lumbar fusions. *Spine* 1989;14(4):358-362.

10. Kobrinsky NL, Letts RM, Patel LR, et al. 1-Deamino-8-D-arginine vasopressin (desmopressin) decreases operative blood loss in patients having Harrington rod spinal fusion surgery: a randomized, double-blinded, controlled trial. *Ann Intern Med* 1987;107(4):446-450.

11. Letts RM. DDAVP (DDAVP): An adjunct to hemostasis? *Spine* 1991;5:103.

12. Menon C, Berry EW, Ockelford P. Beneficial effect of DDAVP on bleeding-time in von Willebrand's disease. *Lancet* 1978;2(8092 Pt 1):743-4. Letter.

13. Czer LS, Bateman TM, Gray RJ, et al. Prospective trial of DDAVP in treatment of severe platelet dysfunction and hemorrhage after cardiopulmonary bypass. *Circulation* 1985;72(suppl 3):130.

14. Hedderich GS, Petsikas DJ, Cooper BA, et al. DDAVP acetate in uncomplicated coronary artery bypass surgery: a prospective randomized clinical trial. *Can J Surg* 1990;33(1):33-36. Comments.

15. Rocha E, Llorens R, Paramo JA, Arcas R, Cuesta B, Trenor AM. Does desmopressin acetate reduce blood loss after surgery in patients on cardiopulmonary bypass? *Circulation* 1988;77(6):1319-1323.

16. Yarom R, Muhlrad A, Hodges S, Robin GC. Platelet pathology in patients with idiopathic scoliosis: Ultrastructural morphometry, aggregations, x-ray spectrometry, and biochemical analysis. *Lab Invest* 1980;43(3):208-216.

17. Lawhon SM, Kahn A III, et al. Controlled hypotensive anaesthesia during spinal surgery: A retrospective study. *Spine* 1984; 9:450-453.

18. Uden A, Nilsson IM, Willner S. Collagen-induced platelet aggregation and bleeding time in adolescent idiopathic scoliosis. *Acta Orthop Scand* 1980;51(5):773-777.

19. Sollevi A. Hypotensive anesthesia and blood loss. *Acta Anaesthesiol Scand* (suppl): 1988;89:39-43.

20. Johnson RG. Blood loss in spinal surgery: prevention and replacement. State of the art reviews. *Spine* 1991;.

21. Tate D Jr, Friedman RJ. Blood conservation in spinal surgery: review of current techniques. *Spine* 1992;17(12):1450-1456.

22. Simpson MB, Georgopoulos G, Eilert RE. Intraoperative blood salvage in children and young adults undergoing spinal surgery with predeposited autologous blood: efficacy and cost-effectiveness. *J Pediatr Orthop* 1993;13(6):777-780.

23. Lawhon SM, Kahn A 3rd, Crawford AH, Brinker MS. Controlled hypotensive anesthesia during spinal surgery: a retrospective study. *Spine* 1984;9(5):450-453.

24. Guay J, Haig M, Lortie L, Guertin MC, Poitras B. Predicting blood loss in surgery for idiopathic scoliosis. *Can J Anaesth* 1994;41(9):775-781.

25. Jacobs HK, Lieponis JV, Bunch WH, Barber MJ, Salem MR. The influence of halothane and nitroprusside on canine spinal cord hemodynamics. *Spine* 1982;7(1):35-40.

26. Hardman E. Blood conservation in major orthopedic surgery. *Orthop Rel Res* 1990;256:299.

27. Blevins FT, Shaw B, Valeri CR, Kasser J, Hall J. Reinfusion of shed blood after orthopaedic procedures in children and adolescents. *J Bone Joint Surg Am* 1993;75(3):363-371.

28. Biesma DH, Kraaijenhagen RJ, Poortman J, Marx JJ, van-de-Wiel A. The effect of oral iron supplementation on erythropoiesis in autologous blood donors. *Transfusion* 1992;32(2):162-165. Comments.

29. Jay J, Flynn JC, Bierman AH. Erythrocyte survival following intraoperative autotransfusion in spine surgery. *Spine* 1986;11:879-882.

Aprotinin Administration in Patients Undergoing Complex Total Hip Arthroplasty

John M. Murkin, MD

Patients undergoing complex total-hip arthroplasty (THA), which includes such procedures as revision or bilateral primary THA, are at increased risk of perioperative complications. This patient population tends to be older, frequently suffering from hypertension, heart disease, and diabetes, as well as degenerative joint disease. The most common life-threatening complications are thromboembolism, myocardial infarction, and congestive heart failure.[1] Blood loss requiring transfusion is another significant factor that influences perioperative morbidity. Blood loss is increased when considerable soft tissue must be released (as in revision THA), when components and cement from the original procedure must be removed, and after more extensive prior surgery, eg, Girdlestone arthroplasty.[1] In addition, these complex procedures take longer, and the duration of surgery has a direct impact on the extent of blood loss.

Some THA procedures may be carried out with less than 500 mL blood loss and require no specific replacement therapy either intraoperatively or postoperatively.[1] Most series reported in the literature, however, demonstrate much higher rates of blood loss. In a series of patients undergoing revision THA, blood loss averaged 2245 mL, and an average of 1160 mL of homologous blood was transfused.[2] Another study reported a 1834 mL blood loss that required an average blood replacement of 1539 mL.[3]

Several recent studies have demonstrated decreased blood loss and transfusion requirements in patients undergoing primary hip arthroplasty and treated with the serine protease inhibitor aprotinin. These studies demonstrated significant reductions in blood loss from 20% to 30% and halved transfusion requirements.[4-6]

However, risk/benefit considerations need to be addressed if hemostatic agents are to be given to the high-risk patient undergoing complex THA. The benefit of improved hemostasis must be considered against the possible increased risk of thrombotic complications.

THROMBOEMBOLIC RISK AFTER THA

Deep-vein thrombosis (DVT) is the most common serious complication after THA and is reported to occur in over 50% of patients who receive no antithrombotic prophylaxis.[7] Deep-vein thrombosis is responsible for the majority of postoperative morbidity after THA and is etiologic in pulmonary embolism (PE), the most common cause of death within 3 months of surgery.[8] Pulmonary embolism occurs in up to 20% of untreated patients after THA, and fatal PE occurs in up to 6%, in contrast to an incidence of fatal PE of 0.1% to 0.8% observed in general surgery patients.[7]

The three primary factors involved in thromboembolism—stasis, tissue injury, and hypercoagulability—can all be identified in the context of THA. Intraoperative phlebography has demonstrated severe distortion and stasis of the femoral vein during surgical manipulation of the operative leg.[9] This likely results in direct endothelial damage and initiation of thrombus formation and may account for the preponderance of DVT occurring at the level of the greater trochanter in the femoral vein of the operative leg, where maximal intraoperative trauma to this vein occurs.[10] The vasoconstrictor response to injury may be lost under certain circumstances during surgery, and intraoperative venodilation and implied endothelial damage from release of humoral substances have been demonstrated in patients undergoing THA and correlated with development of DVT.[11] Intraoperative venoconstrictor therapy with dihydroergotamine in combination with heparin has demonstrated significant reductions in the incidence of DVT and PE.[7] Thrombocytosis and increased platelet adhesiveness have also been documented within the first postoperative day and reflect the stress response to surgical trauma.[12]

APROTININ USE IN THA

As a nonspecific inhibitor of serine proteases, aprotinin binds to various proteolytic enzymes in a dose-dependent manner. A wide variety of serine proteases involved in inflammation and coagulation are inhibited to variable degrees by the concentrations of aprotinin achieved in the plasma with clinical dosages. Activity is measured as kallikrein inhibitory units (KIU). In clinical practice, concentrations of 100 to 200 KIU/mL are achieved. Figure 1 shows the classical coagulation cascade, comprising both the contact activated (intrinsic) pathway and the extrinsic pathway. Aprotinin can inhibit contact activation via its action to inhibit kallikrein, factor XIIa, and factor IXa. Studies in vitro have demonstrated a 20% reduction in factor XIIa activity, a 50% reduction in factor IXa activity, and prolongation of the partial thromboplastin time by a concentration of 200 KIU/mL aprotinin.[13] Thus, in clinical practice, aprotinin has the potential of exerting a significant effect to reduce activation of the coagulation cascade via the intrinsic pathway.

The rationale for using aprotinin in complex THA patients is two-fold: (1) to reduce perioperative blood loss and the need for blood-product transfusion; and (2) to reduce the likelihood of venous thrombosis.

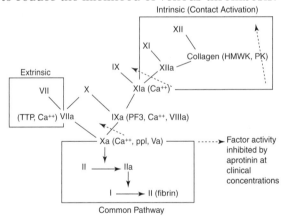

Fig 1. Coagulation cascade comprising both contact activated pathway and extrinsic pathway. Role of clinical concentrations of aprotinin in inhibiting activation through the contact pathway by inhibiting activity of both factor XIIa and factor IXa, as well as inhibiting kallikrein activity, is shown. PK, Prekallikrein; HMWK, high-molecular-weight kininogen. (Reprinted with permission from *Blood Conservation With Aprotinin*. Philadelphia, Pa: Hanley and Belfus Inc; 1995: 373-389.)

Action of Aprotinin in Reducing Blood Loss and Transfusion Requirements

Aprotinin has been shown to decrease blood loss and blood-product transfusion in patients undergoing a variety of cardiac and noncardiac surgical procedures such as liver transplantation and major vascular reconstruction.[14-19] Several recent studies have demonstrated a 20% to 30% reduction in blood loss and significantly lower transfusion requirements in patients undergoing primary THA.[4-6]

Action of Aprotinin in Reducing Venous Thrombosis

Aprotinin's potential for reducing the thromboembolic risk associated with THA relates to its action as a nonspecific serine protease inhibitor. In addition to its actions on intrinsic coagulation activation, aprotinin has been shown to affect the platelet activation that may result from surgical trauma. In orthopedic patients, both collagen-induced platelet aggregability and glass-bead platelet retention have been shown to be significantly decreased by aprotinin.[20] Leukocyte tumor necrosis factor (TNF) and platelet-activating factor (PAF) released as a result of surgical trauma are important mediators of platelet activation and are also both suppressed by aprotinin.[21] Consistent with this, recent clinical data reported by Janssen[5] in patients undergoing primary THA indicate a trend towards a decreased incidence of DVT after aprotinin administration.

Aprotinin in Complex THA

The potential benefits of aprotinin in improving hemostasis without increased risk of thrombotic complications led to a study in a population of high-risk orthopedic patients undergoing complex THA.[22] Patients in this study population were at increased risk of excessive blood loss because of the greater complexity and duration of the surgery.[1] Fifty-three consecutive patients undergoing revision or bilateral primary THA were studied. Patients were assigned to receive either aprotinin or an equivalent volume of saline placebo, administered from uniformly blinded bottles as a continuous infusion for the duration of the surgery and for 1 hour postoperatively. Patients weighing between 60 and 80 kg and randomized to receive aprotinin were given a 2 million KIU (200 mL) loading dose over 15 minutes, followed by an infusion of 0.5 million KIU (50 mL) per hour. Those weighing less than 60 kg or more than 80 kg received a 2.8 mL/kg (10,000 KIU/mL) loading dose and an infusion of 0.7 mL/kg/h. Placebo-treated patients received an equivalent volume of 0.9% saline. The plasma concentration of aprotinin 1 hour after start of surgery was approximately 130 KIU/mL and was similar for both dosage regimens.

To assess the risk of venous thromboembolism developing, patients underwent bilateral compression color Doppler ultrasound of the lower limbs preoperatively and within 7 to 8 days postoperatively. Doppler ultrasound was used rather than venography to enable greater compliance with repeat examination. It was felt important to assess patients preoperatively as well as postoperatively to detect preexisting thrombosis from previous hip-replacement surgery. Compression ultrasound can identify proximal DVT with sufficient accuracy and may be insensitive only to small valve cuff thrombi that are of questionable clinical significance.[23] Patients with abnormal Doppler ultrasound or clinical symptoms of DVT underwent venography. The demographic data for the 29 patients in the aprotinin-treated group and the 24 patients in the placebo control group were comparable for age, weight, gender, and the duration of surgery and hospitalization. The six patients with diabetes were all in the aprotinin group, and this group also had more patients on preoperative aspirin therapy. All patients were treated with antithrombotic prophylaxis (warfarin or heparin) starting the day prior to surgery and continuing until hospital discharge.

Intraoperative blood loss was measured by suction losses and weight of sponges; postoperative losses were determined by the volume of wound drainage until removal of the drains at approximately 48 hours after surgery. Aprotinin-treated patients experienced significantly less postoperative blood loss and approximately 25% overall reduction in total blood loss (the Table). There was no difference between groups in the percentage of patients requiring blood transfusion, but of patients who were transfused, aprotinin-treated patients required less packed red blood cells (the Table). The reduced volume of red cells transfused in the aprotinin-treated patients did not result in postoperative anemia, as both preoperative and postoperative hemoglobin concentrations were similar between groups. The action of aprotinin to inhibit contact activation of the coagulation cascade was confirmed in this study by the prolongation of the activated partial thromboplastin time (aPTT)—a measure of contact activation—in the aprotinin-treated patients.

Blood Loss and Blood-Transfusion Requirements			
	Aprotinin (n = 29)	Control (n = 24)	*P* Value
Intraoperative (mL)	996 ± 81	1318 ± 145	0.060
Postoperative (mL)	502 ± 62	778 ± 118	0.046
Total (mL)	1498 ± 110	2096 ± 223	0.022
Patients transfused	18 (62 1%)	17 (70.8%)	
Transfusion of RBCs (U)	2.0 ± 0.2	2.9 ± 0.4	0.039

Values are mean ± SEM. RBCs, Red blood cells.
(Modified from Murkin JM, Shannon NA, Bourne RB, et al. *Anesthesia Analgesia.* 1995;80:343-348.)

Deep-vein thrombosis was confirmed postoperatively in 3 of 24 patients in the placebo-treated patients, two of whom suffered acute proximal femoral vein thrombosis in the operative limb; one suffered a concomitant postoperative cerebral vascular accident. No DVT was detected in 29 aprotinin-treated patients. Parenthetically, these results for incidence of thromboembolism are similar to those reported in primary hip-replacement surgery.[5] If the results of these two studies are pooled, the incidence of DVT in control groups ranged from 12% to 20%. This is consistent with the average expected incidence of 19% (range 13% to 26%) derived from pooled data on 162 similar patients reported in the literature.[24] In contrast, the incidence of DVT in aprotinin-treated patients was zero in both studies.

SUMMARY

The administration of aprotinin is efficacious in patients undergoing THA, as measured by a decrease in blood loss and lower transfusion requirements. This effect is not contingent on the complexity of the procedure or on whether primary or revision orthopedic hip arthroplasty procedures are undertaken. In addition, aprotinin can be employed without risk of increased thrombotic complications, even in patients at high risk of such events, and studies to date show a trend towards a decreased risk of venous thrombosis in patients treated with aprotinin.

References

1. Harkness J. Arthroplasty of hip. In: Crewshaw A, ed. *Campbell's Operative Orthopedics*. vol 1. St Louis, Mosby Year Book; 1992: 441-626.

2. Wilson WJ. Intraoperative autologous transfusion in revision total hip arthroplasty. *J Bone Joint Surg Am* 1989;71(1):8-14.

3. Woolson ST, Marsh JS, Tanner JB. Transfusion of previously deposited autologous blood for patients undergoing hip-replacement surgery. *J Bone Joint Surg Am* 1987;69(3):325-328.

4. Wollinsky KH, Mehrkens HH, Freytag T, Geiger P, Weindler M. [Does aprotinin lessen intraoperative blood loss?]. *Anasthesiol Intensivmed Notfallmed Schmerzther* 1991;26(4):208-210.

5. Janssens M, Joris J, David JL, Lemaire R, Lamy M. High-dose aprotinin reduces blood loss in patients undergoing total hip replacement surgery *Anesthesiology* 1994;80(1):23-29. Comments.

6. Haas S, Fritsche H, Ritter H, et al. Fuhrt eine perioperative gabe des plasmainhibitors aprotinin zu einer steigerung des postoperativen thromboserisikos? In: Hartel W, Bager H, Ungeheuer, eds. Chirurgisches Forum '91, f. experim. u klinische Forschubg. Berlin, Germany: Springer-Verlag; 1991: 371-374.

7. Haake DA, Berkman SA. Venous thromboembolic disease after hip surgery: risk factors, prophylaxis, and diagnosis. *Clin Orthop* 1989;242:212-231.

8. Johnson R, Green JR, Charnley J. Pulmonary embolism and its prophylaxis following the Charnley total hip replacement. *Clin Orthop* 1977;127:123-132.

9. Stamatakis JD, Kakkar VV, Sagar S, Lawrence D, Nairn D, Bentley PG. Femoral vein thrombosis and total hip replacement. *Br Med J* 1977;2(6081):223-225.

10. Bell WR, Tomasulo PA, Alving BM, Duffy TP. Thrombocytopenia occurring during the administration of heparin: a prospective study in 52 patients. *Ann Intern Med* 1976;85(2):155-160.

11. Stewart G, Ziskin M, Alburger P. Correlation of venous dilation during hip arthroplasty and subsequent development of deep vein thrombosis (DVT): clinical study using intraoperative ultrasound (US) monitoring. *Thromb Haemost* 1985;4:247-250.

12. Bennett PN. Postoperative changes in platelet adhesiveness. *J Clin Pathol* 1967;20(5):708-709.

13. Harke H, Gennrich M. Aprotinin-ACD-blood. I: experimental studies on the effect of aprotinin on the plasmatic and thrombocytic coagulation. *Anaesthesist* 1980;29(5):266-276.

14. Bidstrup B, Harrison J, Royston D. Aprotinin therapy in cardiac operations: a report of use in 41 cardiac centres in the United Kingdom. *Ann Thorac Surg* 1993;55:971-976.

15. Dietrich W, Barankay A, Dilthey G, et al. Reduction of homologous blood requirement in cardiac surgery by intraoperative aprotinin application—clinical experience in 152 cardiac surgical patients. *Thorac Cardiovasc Surg* 1989;37(2):92-98.

16. Royston D, Bidstrup BP, Taylor KM, Sapsford RN. Effect of aprotinin on need for blood transfusion after repeat open-heart surgery. *Lancet* 1987;2(8571):1289-1291.

17. Neuhaus P, Bechstein WO, Lefebre B, Blumhardt G, Slama K. Effect of aprotinin on intraoperative bleeding and fibrinolysis in liver transplantation. *Lancet* 1989;2(8668):924-925. Letter.

18. Mallett SV, Cox D, Burroughs AK, Rolles K. Aprotinin and reduction of blood loss and transfusion requirements in orthotopic liver transplantation. *Lancet* 1990;336(8719):886-887. Letter.

19. Thompson JF, Roath OS, Francis JL, Webster JH, Chant AD. Aprotinin in peripheral vascular surgery. *Lancet* 1990;335(8694):911. Letter.

20. Ketterl R, Haas S, Lechner F, Kienzle H, Blumel G. [Effect of aprotinin on thrombocytic function during total endoprosthesis surgery of the hip]. *Med Welt* 1980;31(35):1239-1243.

21. Hunyadi J, Kenderessy AS, Duda E, Braquet P, Dobozy A. Platelet-activating factor antagonists (BN 52021 and BN 50730) inhibit tumor necrosis factor-alfa-mediated cytotoxicity on murine L929 tumor cells. *Mol Immunol* 1993;30(6):517-519.

22. Murkin JM, Shannon NA, Bourne RB, Rorabeck CH, Cruickshank M, Wyile G. Aprotinin decreases blood loss in patients undergoing revision or bilateral total hip arthroplasty. *Anesth Analg* 1995;80(2):343-348.

23. Cronan JJ. Ultrasound evaluation of deep venous thrombosis. *Semin Roentgenol* 1992;27(1):39-52.

24. Clagett GP, Anderson F Jr, Levine MN, Salzman EW, Wheeler HB. Prevention of venous thromboembolism. *Chest* 1992;102(4 suppl):391S-407S. Comments.

Changing Transfusion Requirements: Guidelines and Decisions

Gary Hartstein, MD

Since the mid-1980s, public awareness of transfusion risks, concerns over adequacy of supply, and cost considerations have led to marked changes in the clinical practice of physicians responsible for transfusing blood products, especially in the perioperative setting.[1] Reduced use of homologous blood, increased reliance on autologous transfusions (obtained either preoperatively or in the operating room itself), and the introduction of pharmacologic tools for reducing blood loss are the results of these changes. Because of a notable paucity of controlled studies, guidelines designed to help clinical decision-making have been formulated.[2] As knowledge of the pathophysiology of acute anemia increases, these guidelines must be continually reviewed and should be updated as new data become available.

In addition to increased emphasis on reducing blood loss and on using the patient's own blood, setting a lower level of hemoglobin and hematocrit is another way of decreasing reliance on homologous blood. The theoretical background and clinical approach pertaining to a lower transfusion trigger form the basis of this chapter.

Before ordering transfusion of red blood cells (RBCs), the clinician must implicitly or explicitly ask three questions: First, *why* transfuse? The answer requires an understanding of oxygen delivery to the tissues and of the compensatory mechanisms used by the organism to cope with acute anemia. The second question is *when*? Here, the physician must use skill and knowledge to determine when the limits of compensation have been reached for a given patient. The different sensitivities of various organ systems to anemia, as well as the effects of coexisting pathologies on these sensitivities, should be factored into this decision. Finally, we must ask *how* best to transfuse. Practical aspects of transfusion therapy itself, as well as medicolegal considerations, are best dealt with under this heading. A clear enumeration of reasons NOT to transfuse also should be reviewed.

WHY TRANSFUSE?

The only reason to consider transfusing RBCs is to increase the oxygen-carrying capacity of the blood and, consequently, the delivery of oxygen to tissues. The oxygen content of arterial blood (C_aO_2) consists almost entirely of oxygen bound to hemoglobin, with a small amount dissolved in the plasma. The formula below shows that when the oxyhemoglobin saturation (S_aO_2) is within normal limits, oxygen content depends on the hemoglobin (Hb) concentration:

$$C_aO_2 = (Hb \times 1.34) \times S_aO_2 + (0.0031 \times P_aO_2)$$

It should be clear that any reduction in circulating hemoglobin concentration will produce an immediate proportional reduction in the arterial oxygen content. When arterial oxygen content is multiplied by cardiac output (Q_t), the result is the amount of oxygen delivered to the tissues (DO_2):

$$DO_2 = C_aO_2 \times Q_t$$

Under normal conditions, the delivery of oxygen to the body's tissues is about four times greater than the amount consumed. This implies a considerable reserve in terms of the supply/demand ratio. The ratio of total-body oxygen consumption (VO_2) to oxygen delivery is called the oxygen extraction ratio (OER):

$$OER = VO_2/DO_2 \text{ (normal 25\%)}$$

Compensatory Mechanisms

Reduction in levels of hemoglobin call into play certain compensatory mechanisms to maintain adequate oxygen supply to the tissues. Two principal types of compensation are seen: increased cardiac output and increased off-loading of oxygen from hemoglobin at the tissue level.

Increased Cardiac Output

Increased venous return to the heart is the primary factor in the increased cardiac output seen in (normovolemic) anemic patients. In addition, the impedance to cardiac ejection decreases, as a result of both decreased blood viscosity and peripheral vasodilation. These effects combine to increase stroke volume. It should be noted that despite higher ejected volumes, myocardial work does not increase when only these mechanisms are operant. On the other hand, when the degree of anemia is severe and/or in patients unable to modulate their stroke volume, the energetically less favorable mechanisms of increased contractility and tachycardia (both induced by stimulation of the sympathetic nervous system) become necessary.

Increased Oxygen Extraction

A number of factors contribute to increased off-loading of oxygen from hemoglobin at the level of tissues. These include capillary recruitment and a rightward shift of the hemoglobin-oxygen dissociation curve. The Bohr effect is responsible for this shift in the acute situation, while increased intraerythrocytic levels of 2,3-diphosphoglycerate acid (2,3 DPG) become operant over 48 to 72 hours.

WHEN TO TRANSFUSE

As a result of the above compensatory mechanisms, and provided normovolemia is strictly maintained, oxygen supply to the tissues of healthy subjects remains normal until the hematocrit falls below 30%.[3] Levels of hemoglobin considerably lower than this can often be tolerated. However, the ability to tolerate such degrees of hemodilution will vary considerably among patient populations.

Tolerance of Anemia

Good clinical data are scarce in the literature, but evidence from animal studies suggests that very low hematocrits can be tolerated in healthy individuals. A study in baboons hemodiluted to a hematocrit of 15% and subjected to surgical stress (a laparotomy) showed no morbidity after a 2-month follow-up period.[4] A further study in anesthetized dogs hemodiluted to a hematocrit of 22% demonstrated preservation of both myocardial and cerebral perfusion under these circumstances.[5] Table 1 shows some of the limited data available from human studies, most of which consist of clinical series.[6-10]

Table 1. Clinical Studies on Tolerance of Anemia in Various Patient Populations

Study Outcome	Threshold	Population	Clinical
Fullerton & Turner[6]	> 45 g/L	Pregnant women with malaria	ND, NCF
Gollub & Bailey[7]	> 70 g/L	Cardiac surgery— Jehovah's Witnesses	NC
Alexiu et al[8]	> 50 g/L	Surgery— bleeding ulcers	NC
Kawaguchi et al[9]	> 70 g/L	Pediatric cardiac surgery	ND
Carson et al[10]	> 80 g/L	Surgery— Jehovah's Witnesses	ND

ND, no deaths; NCF, no cardiac failure; NC, no complications.

While no firm data are yet available detailing when to initiate RBC transfusion, useful suggestions can be made. A Consensus Conference on Perioperative Red Blood Cell Transfusion suggested that "otherwise healthy patients with hemoglobin values of 100 g/L or greater rarely require perioperative transfusion, whereas those with acute anemia ... less than 70 g/L frequently will require red cell transfusions."[2] The American Association of Blood Banks uses 80 g/L as a lower limit.

An important question to address is whether this lower limit can be applied to all patient populations. In particular, the effects of age and concomitant diseases both on peripheral oxygen requirements and on the capacity to adapt to anemia must be kept in mind when deciding the need to increase red-cell mass by transfusion.

Coronary Artery Disease and Tolerance of Anemia

Because oxygen extraction across the capillary bed of the heart is maximal even under basal conditions, any increase in myocardial oxygen demand must be met by an increase in nutritive flow, itself dependent on a vasodilatory response. The heart is thus considered to be the organ most at risk for decreased blood oxygen-carrying capacity. The patient with coronary artery disease therefore deserves special attention when considering the limits of tolerance of anemia.

Data from animal experimentation support the view that the compromised myocardium is less able to tolerate anemia. Rats in whom coronary ligation led to myocardial infarction (as opposed to those in whom similar ligation did not lead to cellular necrosis) were unable to compensate for a moderate hemodilution (to 30%) by an increase in cardiac output.[11] Crystal selectively perfused the left anterior descending artery of anesthetized dogs; with graded hemodilution, it was observed that once coronary vasodilator reserve was exhausted, myocardial ischemia became very prominent.[12] There is additional evidence that animals with myocardial depression cannot respond appropriately to hemodilution.[13]

There are human data on the influence of hemodilution on myocardial ischemia. A study in high-risk (ASA class III) patients undergoing vascular surgery showed that new episodes of ischemia (diagnosed using Holter ST-segment monitoring) occurred in 55% of patients with a hematocrit below 29% compared with only 16% in patients with a hematocrit above 29%. The effects were most noticeable on the first and second postoperative days.[14] Very similar results were found, again in vascular surgery patients, with only two of 14 patients with a hematocrit above 28% showing ischemic changes postoperatively, compared with 10 out of 13 with values less than 28%. There were six morbid events, defined as acute pulmonary edema, arrhythmias, or myocardial infarctions.[15] The study by Singbartl et al[16] in patients undergoing orthopedic surgery with hemodilution found similar incidences of ischemic events between healthy (ASA I and II) and sicker (ASA III) patients. However, the hemoglobin levels were significantly higher in the sicker patients, 63 g/L versus 47 g/L, again reinforcing the notion that tolerance of anemia is strongly influenced by the physical condition of the patient.

One report involving patients with coronary artery disease having aortic reconstructions suggested a lower incidence of ischemia (diagnosed with transesophageal echocardiography) with lower hematocrits. This was explained by the beneficial effects of reduced viscosity and improved local blood flow. In addition, these patients were not severely hemodiluted.[17]

Another situation often encountered when blood loss is to be reduced is controlled hypotension. Use of this technique could conceivably impact on compensatory mechanisms for concomitant hemodilution. Animal data suggest increased aortic and myocardial blood flows and well-preserved myocardial oxygen supply and demand when dogs were hemodiluted to a hematocrit of 22%. However, when hypotension was then induced with adenosine, oxygen deficit occurred in all organs except for the heart. It is highly likely that the heart was protected, in this study, by the beneficial actions of adenosine on the myocardium; this may not have been the case if hypotension had been induced using another agent.[5]

There are certainly other high-risk patient populations with impaired capabilities to compensate for anemia. Although good clinical data are lacking, these populations probably include patients with valvular heart disease, cerebrovascular disease, and pulmonary disease, as well as the elderly, and patients taking beta blockers.

HOW TO TRANSFUSE
As mentioned above, the only reason to transfuse RBCs is to maintain an adequate supply of oxygen to the tissues. Transfusions should NOT be given to promote wound healing, to avoid postoperative infections, or to enhance a sense of well-being. Red-cell transfusion should never be performed to increase the intravascular volume.

Normovolemia should be aggressively established with the use of clear fluids. Normal circulating volume serves several purposes in the presence of anemia. It allows full exploitation of compensatory mechanisms. Symptoms of hypoperfusion due to inadequate fluid replacement can thus be distinguished from those due to inadequate oxygen carriage. Finally, once the circulating mass has been restored, the true values of hemoglobin and hematocrit can be obtained.

Clinical decision-making should begin preoperatively. Patients likely to tolerate low levels of hemoglobin, as well as those probably at risk for normovolemic anemia, can be identified based on their history, physical examination, and laboratory investigations. When assessing patients at high risk, it should be remembered that approximately two-thirds of myocardial ischemic events are clinically silent. If an aggressive policy of blood conservation is to be applied, it may be necessary to pursue a policy of preoperative and intraoperative monitoring using, for example, Holter ST-segment analysis (preoperatively) or continuous ST-segment monitoring (intraoperatively) to identify patients with overt or covert coronary artery disease. Intraoperative decisions to transfuse, and the transfusion trigger to be used, can then be based on the assessed distinction between low-risk and high-risk patients.

Intraoperatively, following trends in automatically recorded ST segments may be useful during progressive hemodilution in high-risk patients. Measurement of mixed-venous oxygen saturation (which requires catheterization of the pulmonary artery) can be invaluable in assessing the balance between myocardial oxygen supply and demand. When the OER exceeds 50%, the myocardium begins to produce lactate, indicative of ischemia.[18]

Postoperatively, it must be remembered that the patient's oxygen demands will increase. Signs and symptoms of anemia must be sought, which include dyspnea, normovolemic orthostatism, tachycardia, evidence of myocardial or cerebral ischemia, and syncope. The increased incidence of silent myocardial ischemia in the postoperative period should be remembered.[19]

Once the decision to transfuse has been made, it should proceed on a unit-by-unit basis. Old dogma dictating multiple-unit transfusions no longer holds. Reevaluation should precede administration of each subsequent unit.

PRACTICAL GUIDELINES
- Establish and verify normovolemia.
- Remember differences in the reference ranges of hemoglobin between genders (males 136 g/L; females 120 g/L) when the transfusion trigger is decided upon.
- Consider the high-risk versus low-risk patients on an individual basis.
- When blood loss is massive and ongoing, TRANSFUSE.
- If aggressive blood-conservation policy with hemodilution is to be used, consider aggressive monitoring in high-risk patients.
- Address issues related to informed consent. Discuss the risks and benefits of and alternatives to homologous blood with the patient and surgeon PRIOR to surgery.

References

1. Heaton W. Changing patterns of blood use. *Transfusion* 1994;34:365-367. Editorial.

2. Consensus Conference. Perioperative red blood cell transfusion. *JAMA* 1988;260:2700-2703.

3. Van der Linden P. The optimal hematocrit. In: Vincent JL, ed. *Update in Critical Care and Emergency Medicine.* 1994:227-236.

4. Levine E, Rosen A, Sehgal L, et al. Physiologic effects of acute anemia: implications for a reduced transfusion trigger. *Transfusion* 1990;30:11-14.

5. Crystal GJ, Rooney MW, Salem MR. Regional hemodynamics and oxygen supply during isovolemic hemodilution alone and in combination with adenosine-induced controlled hypotension. *Anesth Analg* 1988;67:211-218.

6. Fullerton WT, Turner AG. Exchange transfusion in treatment of severe anemia in pregnancy. *Lancet* 1962;1:75-78.

7. Gollub S, Bailey CP. Management of major surgical blood loss without transfusion. *JAMA* 1966;198:149-152.

8. Alexiu O, Mircea N, Balabar M, et al. Gastrointestinal hemorrhage from peptic ulcer: an evaluation of bloodless transfusion and early surgery. *Anaesthesia* 1975;30:609-615.

9. Kawaguchi A, Bergsland J, Subramanian S. Total bloodless open heart surgery in the pediatric age group. *Circulation* 1984;70(3 pt 2):130-137.

10. Carson JL, Poses RM, Spence RK, et al. Severity of anaemia and operative mortality and morbidity. *Lancet* 1988;1:727-729.

11. Kobayashi H, Estafanous FG, Fouad FM. Effects of myocardial infaction on hemodynamic responses to variable degrees of hemodilution. *Anesth Analg* 1988;67:5117. Abstract.

12. Crystal GJ. Coronary hemodynamic responses during local hemodilution in canine hearts. *Am J Physiol* 1988;254:H525-531.

13. Estafanous FG, Smith CE, Selim WM, et al. Cardiovascular effects of acute normovolemic hemodilution in rats with disopyramide-induced myocardial depression. *Basic Res Cardiol* 1990;85:227-236.

14. Christopherson R, Frank S, Norris E, et al. Low postoperative hematocrit is associated with cardiac ischemia in high-risk patients. *Anesthesiology* 1991;75:A99. Abstract.

15. Nelson AH, Fleisher LA, Rosenbaum SH. Relationship between postoperative anemia and cardiac morbidity in high-risk vascular patients in the intensive care unit. *Crit Care Med* 1993;21:860-866.

16. Singbartl G, Becker M, Frankenberg C, et al. Intraoperative on-line ST segment analysis with extreme normovolemic hemodilution. *Anesth Analg* 1992;74:S295. Abstract.

17. Catoire P, Saada M, Gormenzano G, et al. Evaluation of the effects of preoperative normovolemic hemodilution by TEE in coronary artery disease patients. *Anesthesiology* 1991;75:A106. Abstract.

18. Wilkerson DK, Rosen AL, Gould S, et al. Oxygen extraction ratio: a valid indicator of myocardial metabolism in anemia. *J Surg Res* 1987;42:629-634.

19. Mangano DT, Hollenberg M, Feyert G, et al. Perioperative myocardial ischemia in patients undergoing noncardiac surgery: incidence and severity during the four-day perioperative period. *J Am Coll Cardiol* 1991;17:843-850.

Effects of Pharmacologic Intervention in Patients Undergoing Total Hip Replacement

Sylvia Haas, MD

Total hip replacement is associated with significant tissue trauma, and the mechanical processes involved in inserting the prosthesis can lead to the release of particles of bone marrow, fat, and cement. Transesophageal echocardiographic (TEE) monitoring of the right atrium will demonstrate major and minor particles associated with implantation of the femoral shaft and the use of methylmethacrylate cement. This leads to the initiation of a biochemical cascade of events involving activation of the coagulation and fibrinolytic systems and activation of blood platelets.[1,2] Derangement of hemostasis and homeostasis produces clinical complications of excess bleeding and increased thrombotic risk.

ACTION OF APROTININ ON PLATELET FUNCTION

Platelets play a specific role in perioperative bleeding complications, and the ability to influence their activation during complex orthopedic surgery is of great clinical importance. The serine protease inhibitor aprotinin (Bayer, Leverkusen, Germany) has been shown to have a stabilizing effect on platelets in vitro.[3,4] These laboratory studies led us to perform a series of clinical trials to investigate platelet function in patients undergoing major bone surgery, some of whom were treated with aprotinin at the beginning of surgery. Two groups of patients given 20,000 KIU/kg body-weight aprotinin and 10,000 KIU/kg body-weight aprotinin were compared with a control group of patients.[5] The aprotinin dose was based on results obtained from in vitro experiments and was less than the recommended dose that was published several years later in 1987 when the blood-sparing action of aprotinin was first investigated.[6]

Citrated blood was drawn at various times up to 2 hours after aprotinin treatment. Platelet adhesiveness was evaluated by measuring platelet retention on unsiliconized glass beads.[7] The in vitro action of aprotinin was assessed by incubating blood with 200 KIU/mL or 100 KIU/mL aprotinin for 20 minutes at 37°C. These samples were obtained from patients prior to aprotinin administration.

Platelet adhesion was significantly increased in the saline control group, whereas a significant decrease was seen after treatment with aprotinin. The higher-dose aprotinin was more effective. A dose-dependent decrease in platelet adhesiveness was also seen with the in vitro incubation of patient blood with aprotinin (Fig 1).

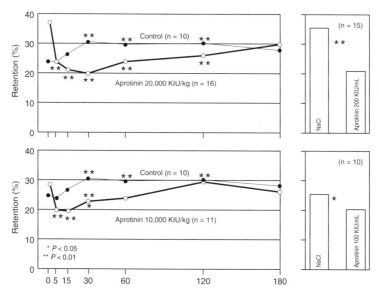

Fig 1. Platelet adhesion in major bone surgery (left) compared with initial value. In vitro incubations (right). (Reprinted with permission from Pa, Pifarré R, ed. *Blood Conservation With Aprotinin*. Philadelphia, Pa: Hanley & Belfus; 1995:103-129.)

A further study was performed in patients undergoing alloarthroplastic total hip replacement with cemented femoral prostheses and treated with 20,000 KIU/kg body-weight aprotinin at the start of surgery. The results confirmed our first study, with platelet retention on glass beads peaking at the time of the preparation of the femoral shaft and indicating an increase in platelet reactivity in vivo. In contrast, the group of patients treated with aprotinin showed a significant decrease in platelet adhesion that persisted throughout the surgical period. The ratio of platelet aggregates, which indicates the amount of circulating aggregates, is shown in Fig 2. If no aggregates were present, the ratio would be 1; a ratio of 0 would indicate that all the circulating platelets were aggregated. The normal ratio is between 0.8 and 1. The placebo group showed a significantly higher level of circulating aggregates, whereas the opposite was seen in the aprotinin-treated patients. Platelet aggregation induced by adenosine diphosphate (ADP), collagen, and epinephrine was also significantly reduced in the aprotinin group.[8]

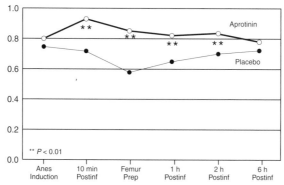

Fig 2. Ratio of platelet aggregates in total-hip replacement. (Reprinted with permission from Pa, Pifarré R, ed. *Blood Conservation With Aprotinin*. Philadelphia, Pa: Hanley & Belfus; 1995:103-129.)

APROTININ AND DEEP-VEIN THROMBOSIS

Deep-vein thrombosis (DVT) occurs in 60% to 70% of patients undergoing surgery for total hip replacement[9] and up to 40% of patients treated with heparin prophylaxis. This may be in part because fibrinolytic activity is decreased or inhibited after major surgical procedures. Thus it is of great clinical interest to determine whether perioperative administration of aprotinin is associated with an increased risk of DVT, particularly in patients at high risk of thromboembolic complications despite prophylaxis with low-dose heparin. To answer this question, a randomized, double-blind, parallel-group trial was conducted in 1983.[10,11]

One hundred and twenty patients scheduled for elective hip-replacement surgery (with cement implantation; no revision procedures) were enrolled into the study. All patients received 5000 IU of heparin (bid) for routine DVT prophylaxis in a fixed combination with 0.5 mg dihydroergotamine. Within 15 minutes after induction of anesthesia, 150 mL of aprotinin (1.5 million KIU) was administered to the treatment group and 150 mL of saline to the control group. Blood loss and transfusion requirements were determined intraoperatively and postoperatively. The number of patients with reduced hemoglobin (< 10 gm/dL) and wound hematomas was also determined postoperatively. Deep-vein thrombosis was diagnosed by the radio-labeled fibrinogen uptake test (RFUT), which was performed daily until 7 days postoperatively at each of 11 measuring points on the lower extremities. All data were recorded with electronic data processing that enabled the results to be analyzed using two different algorithms to avoid any artifact in the statistical evaluation and any false interpretation of the results.

The table shows the incidence of thrombosis in the two groups analyzed using the two versions of the data-handling algorithms. The results show no significant difference in the frequency of thrombosis between patients in the control group and those treated with aprotinin.

Frequency of Thrombosis			
Version	Thrombosis	Aprotinin n(%)	Placebo n(%)
V1	Yes	25 (45)	20 (38)
	No	30 (55)	32 (62)
V2	Yes	15 (27)	15 (29)
	No	40 (73)	37 (71)
Total		**55**	**52**

Deep-vein thrombosis diagnosed by radio-labeled fibrinogen uptake test (RFUT) performed daily at each of 11 measuring points on the lower extremities. In version 1, the assessment points 0 (area of the groin) on both legs and 0-2 on the operated leg were omitted from the evaluation to exclude nonspecific results due to accumulation of radioactivity in the bladder or wound hematoma. In version 2, the mean value of two adjacent measuring points was used as the basis for the evaluation to ensure that artifacts were excluded. (Reprinted with permission from Pa, Pifarré R, ed. *Blood Conservation With Aprotinin.* Philadelphia, Pa: Hanley & Belfus; 1995:103-129.)

In the aprotinin-treated group, 7 patients (12%) received transfusions, 3 intraoperatively and 4 postoperatively. In comparison, the frequency in the placebo group was significantly higher ($P < 0.01$): 19 patients (32%) received transfusions, 1 intraoperatively and 18 postoperatively. In the aprotinin-treated group, 8 patients (13%) had a postoperative reduction in hemoglobin < 10 gm/dL, compared with 22 patients (38%) in the placebo group. This difference was statistically significant ($P < 0.01$). The number of wound hematomas (15% vs 28%) and the postoperative drainage volumes (580 mL vs 800 mL) were also significantly lower in the aprotinin-treated group ($P < 0.05$) than in the placebo group.

The discovery that aprotinin shows remarkable efficacy in reducing bleeding and the need for blood transfusion was purely by chance; the study design was intended to address prothrombotic concerns. Aprotinin's action on hemostasis is most striking in the postoperative period, despite the fact that treatment was restricted to a single dose at the start of surgery.

The action of aprotinin in inhibiting activation of the intrinsic coagulation system was confirmed with marked elevation in the activated partial thromboplastin time (aPTT) during the operative period. The effect is short-lived, and values are normal by the first postoperative day. These data are of clinical significance to the practicing anesthetist, who should realize that this increase in aPTT is a normal response in patients treated with aprotinin and should not be corrected.

Intraoperative fibrinolysis was also inhibited in the aprotinin-treated patients compared with the placebo group, as evidenced by decreased euglobulin lysis on fibrin plates (Fig 3). Once again this action was short-lived, with no significant difference between the two groups in the postoperative period. Antiplasmin levels were also higher intraoperatively in the aprotinin-treated group, whereas there were no differences in antithrombin III (AT-III) or fibrinogen concentrations (Fig 4).

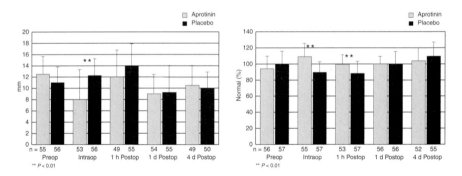

Fig 3. A, Euglobulin lysis on fibrin plates during the perioperative and postoperative periods; B, antiplasmin levels during the perioperative and postoperative periods.

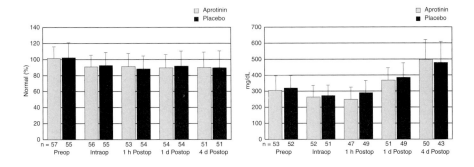

Fig 4. A, Antithrombin III (AT-III) levels during the perioperative and postoperative periods; B, fibrinogen levels during the perioperative and postoperative periods.

The short duration of effect of aprotinin on the parameters measured reflects the short half-life of aprotinin in the plasma. Plasma concentrations measured intraoperatively reached a mean value of 90 KIU/mL during surgery and less than 40 KIU/mL within 1 hour postoperatively. By the first postoperative day, only very low levels were detected.

The biochemical indices measured showed evidence of hypofibrinolysis in the postoperative period. Euglobulin lysis of fibrin plates was markedly reduced on both the first and fourth postoperative days, and the acute-phase reactant proteins antiplasmin and particularly fibrinogen showed significant increases in the postoperative period (Figs 3 and 4,B). These changes indicate an increased thrombogenic risk during this period, and the early perioperative aprotinin therapy did not influence this risk.

Studies of Aprotinin in Orthopedic and Non-Orthopedic Surgery. Our chance finding that aprotinin reduced blood loss and transfusion requirements in patients undergoing hip replacement was confirmed by another piece of serendipity in 1987, this time in patients undergoing cardiac surgery. A study designed to investigate the action of aprotinin in attenuating the inflammatory response of cardiopulmonary bypass demonstrated significant reduction in perioperative bleeding and blood-transfusion requirements.[12] These patients were given a substantially higher dose of aprotinin than had been previously used. Numerous studies have subsequently demonstrated the efficacy of aprotinin as a blood-saving agent in cardiac as well as other types of surgery associated with an increased risk of bleeding.[12-16]

Our early observations of aprotinin's action in reducing perioperative blood loss in orthopedic surgery were confirmed recently by other groups using different dosage regimens. The study from Belgium by Janssens et al[17] used the high-dose regimen described by Royston in 1987: 2 million KIU at the start of surgery, followed by an infusion of half a million KIU throughout the perioperative period.[6] Aprotinin reduced total blood loss from 1943 ± 700 mL to 1446 ± 514 mL ($P < 0.05$). This reduction occurred during surgery ($P < 0.05$) and in the first 5 hours postoperatively ($P < 0.001$). Total amounts of blood transfused were 3.4 ± 1.3 U/patient in the control group and 1.8 ± 1.2 U/patient in the aprotinin group ($P < 0.001$). Despite receiving less transfused packed red cells, aprotinin-treated patients had significantly higher hematocrit on postoperative day 1 and it remained elevated up to day 7. The subjective assessment by the surgeon of bleeding intensity supported the blood-loss data, with no patients in the aprotinin group assessed to have very severe bleeding compared with 5 in the control group.

Two further trials that investigated the efficacy of aprotinin in patients undergoing total hip replacement have been reported. Wollinsky et al, from Germany, found significant reductions in postoperative blood loss (1578 mL vs 1952 mL) in aprotinin-treated patients and placebo-controlled patients, respectively.[18] Ullrich et al, also from Germany, reported similar findings of the efficacy of aprotinin in reducing intraoperative and postoperative blood loss and red blood cell transfusion.[19]

SUMMARY

Perioperative administration of aprotinin reduces both blood loss and blood-product transfusion requirements in patients undergoing total hip replacement. Our results indicate that this is achieved without increasing the risk of postoperative thrombosis. The postoperative period is associated with a hypofibrinolytic state in patients undergoing total hip replacement, with maximal inhibition occurring postoperative days 3 and 4, probably as a result of the concomitant rise in the acute-phase reactant antiplasmin caused by surgical trauma.[11] Aprotinin has a short half-life, and the data available indicate that it does not interfere with this postoperative shutdown of fibrinolysis. It should not, however, be given in the early postoperative period until safety data are available.

The mode of action of aprotinin as a blood-sparing agent in clinical practice is still unclear. There are several possible mechanisms, including inhibition of the intrinsic coagulation pathway via inhibition of kallikrein, modification of platelet function, and/or inhibition of plasmin. In addition, the optimal dose of aprotinin has not been determined.

References

1.   Haas S, Ketterl R, Stemberger A, et al. The effect of aprotinin on platelet function, blood coagulation, and blood lactate level in total hip replacement: a double-blind clinical trial. In: Hörl W, Heidland A, eds. *Protease - Potential Role in Health and Disease.* New York, NY: Plenum Press; 1984:287-297.

2.   Haas S, Ketterl R, Landauer B, et al. Platelet function and proteinase inhibition. In: McConn R, ed. *The Role of Chemical Mediators in the Pathophysiology of Acute Illness and Injury.* New York, NY: Raven Press; 1982:219-228.

3.   Harke H. [Prevention of microaggregation in stored blood (author's trans)]. *Anaesthesist* 1976;25:374-379.

4.   Haas-Denk S, Kaunzner W, Sommoggy Sv. Effects of acetyl-salicylic acid and aprotinin on platelet function and coagulation in stored blood. *Med Welt* 1977;28:912-914.

5.   Ketterl R, Haas S, Lechner F, Kienzle H, Blumel G. [Effect of aprotinin on thrombocytic function during total endoprosthesis surgery of the hip]. *Med Welt* 1980;31:1239-1243.

6.   Royston D, Bidstrup BP, Taylor KM, Sapsford RN. Effect of aprotinin on need for blood transfusion after repeat open-heart surgery. *Lancet* 1987;2:1289-1291.

7.   Morris C. Observations on the effect of glass beads on platelet aggregation and its relation to platelet stickiness. *Thromb Diathes Haemorrh* 1968;20:345.

8.   Haas S, Blumel G. Effect of aprotinin on bleeding complications in noncardiac surgery: experimental studies and clinical trials. In: Pifarré R, ed. *Blood Conservation With Aprotinin.* Philadelphia, Pa: Hanley & Belfus; 1995:103-129.

9. Haake DA, Berkman SA. Venous thromboembolic disease after hip surgery: risk factors, prophylaxis, and diagnosis. *Clin Orthop* 1989;242:212-231.

10. Haas S, Müller-Esterl W, Fritsche H-M, et al. Effect of aprotinin on the incidence of thrombosis and postoperative bleeding. *Thromb Haemost* 1985;54:99.

11. Haas S, Fritsche H-M, Ritter H, et al. Is the risk of postoperative thrombosis increased after perioperative therapy with the plasmin inhibitor aprotinin? In: Hartel Wi et al. ed. *Chirurgisches Forum 1991 für Experimentelle und Klinische. Forschung* Berlin-Heidelberg, Germany: Springer; 1991:371-374.

12. Royston D. The serine antiprotease aprotinin (Trasylol): a novel approach to reducing postoperative bleeding. *Blood Coag Fibrinolys* 1990;1:55-69.

13. Thompson JF, Roath OS, Francis JL, Webster JH, Chant AD. Aprotinin in peripheral vascular surgery. *Lancet* 1990;335:911. Letter.

14. Mallett SV, Cox D, Burroughs AK, Rolles K. Aprotinin and reduction of blood loss and transfusion requirements in orthotopic liver transplantation. *Lancet* 1990;336:886-887. Letter.

15. Bidstrup B, Harrison J, Royston D. Aprotinin therapy in cardiac operations: a report of use in 41 cardiac centres in the United Kingdom. *Ann Thorac Surg* 1993;55:971-976.

16. Neuhaus P, Bechstein WO, Lefebre B, Blumhardt G, Slama K. Effect of aprotinin on intraoperative bleeding and fibrinolysis in liver transplantation. *Lancet* 1989;2:924-925. Letter.

17. Janssens M, Joris J, David JL, Lemaire R, Lamy M. High-dose aprotinin reduces blood loss in patients undergoing total hip replacement surgery. *Anesthesiology* 1994;80:23-29. Comments.

18. Wollinsky KH, Mehrkens HH, Freytag T, Geiger P, Weindler M. [Does aprotinin lessen intraoperative blood loss?]. *Anasthesiol Intensivmed Notfallmed Schmerzther* 1991;26:208-210.

19. Ullrich W, Holz U, Krier C. [Total hip endoprostheses—characteristic aspects from the anesthesiologic viewpoint.] *Anasthesiol Intensivmed Notfallmed Schmerzther* 1994;29:385-399. Comments.

Workshop II:
Blood Conservation
in Transplant Surgery

Pathophysiology of Perioperative Bleeding in Transplant Surgery

R. Patrick Wood, MD, FACS

The number of transplants performed in the United States has increased steadily over the last decade, with about 18,500 performed in 1994 (Table l). The availability of cadaveric organ donors is the rate-limiting factor in all transplantations. The number of organ donors has increased only minimally compared with the number of transplants performed over the last several years. This indicates that more donors are making multiorgan donations.

Table 1. Number of Transplants by Organ, 1987-1993							
	1987	**1988**	**1989**	**1990**	**1991**	**1992**	**1993**
Heart	1438	1663	1700	2085	2126	2173	2290
Heart-lung	49	74	68	50	51	48	60
Kidney	9094	9004	8706	9560	10054	10108	10850
Liver	1199	1711	2164	2656	2953	3056	3441
Lung	0	33	119	262	404	535	658
Pancreas	142	250	419	549	532	555	769
Total	11,922	12,735	13,176	15,162	16,120	16,475	18,068

The scarcity of donor organs causes many patients, especially those in the liver, heart, and lung transplant populations, to wait ever longer for their transplants. Almost 3000 patients died in 1993 while on the transplant waiting list (Fig 1), and the number continues to increase each year. Currently, about 8% of liver transplant candidates will die for want of a donor organ. Another consequence of organ scarcity is that many patients who may have been good transplant candidates when first referred have deteriorated into relatively poor candidates while on the waiting list for a year or more. The morbidity associated with transplantation in these patients is much higher than in good transplant candidates, and the risk of intraoperative bleeding certainly is much greater.

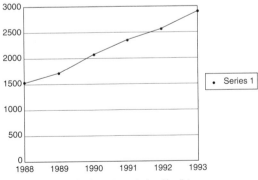

Fig 1. Total deaths on transplant waiting list.

It has long been said that there are two basic tenets in surgical bleeding, particularly that associated with liver transplantation. The first is that the only two types of bleeding to be concerned about is the bleeding you can hear and the bleeding you are standing in. The other is that all bleeding stops eventually. I often retell the story of an incident that occurred in the early days of liver transplantation when a 200-unit blood loss was not uncommon. One day the anesthesiologist walked into the operating room with an armful of blood and blood products and asked the transplant surgeon if he wanted him to give it to the patient or just dump it directly on the floor.

Factors that influence perioperative bleeding in all organ transplants include general condition of the patient, coexisting diseases, prior surgical procedures, retransplantation, and infection. An end-stage patient obviously is at greater risk for perioperative hemorrhage than a patient who is in reasonably good condition. Coexisting diseases, especially liver disease in a patient who is not undergoing liver transplant but rather is receiving a cardiac, pulmonary, or renal transplant, can complicate the perioperative management of coagulation. Adhesions resulting from prior surgical procedures make the technical performance of the operation much more difficult and the risk of massive bleeding much greater. The removal of prior portacaval shunts or multiple prior procedures on the biliary tract can become technically very challenging and blood loss can be surprisingly rapid. During retransplants, and especially orthotopic retransplants, the removal of the old organ and its replacement with a new one present special challenges. Also, patients who are infected may be much more likely to develop disseminated intravascular coagulation (DIC) and other complications with coagulation.

Renal and heart transplants are associated with other specific factors that may affect perioperative bleeding. In renal transplantation, platelet dysfunction due to uremia may be a significant cause of perioperative bleeding. On occasion, a heparin effect may remain in a recently dialyzed patient, particularly if dialyzed directly before coming to the operating room. However, these problems can be addressed relatively easily. A cardiac patient receiving a heart transplant, a heart and lung transplant, or single or double lung transplant may have platelet dysfunction from bypass or heparinization. The management of these problems in the cardiac patient was addressed in earlier presentations.

The challenge of perioperative bleeding is greatest in liver transplants.[1-6] Liver disease has a multitude of effects on hemostasis (Table 2).[7-12] Liver transplant patients may have chronic liver disease or fulminant liver failure. Patients with either chronic or acute liver disease may have decreased synthesis of proteins, including those involved with the coagulation and anticoagulation systems and the pro- and antifibrinolytic systems. Patients with chronic liver disease may synthesize abnormal proteins,[13] including nonfunctional precursors of vitamin K, abnormal factor VIII and von Willebrand factor, and fibrinogen with defective polymerization.[14-18] There is decreased clearance of activated clotting factors, plasminogen activators,[19] and the thrombin-antithrombin complexes produced during the clotting cascade in patients with chronic liver disease.[20] There are platelet abnormalities, with platelets both decreased in number and impaired in their ability to aggregate. Patients with portal hypertension often have thrombocytopenia induced by hypersplenism.

Table 2. Effects of Liver Disease on Hemostasis

Decreased synthesis of proteins
    Coagulation: FXII, XI, IX, VII, V,
                            11 fibrinogen, prekallikrein,
                            kininogen

    Anticoagulant: Proteins C and S,
                            Antithrombin III

    Profibrinolytic: Plasminogen

    Antifibrinolytic: α_2-antiplasmin,
                            C1-inhibitor, α_2-macroglobulin
                            Histidine-rich glycoprotein

Synthesis of abnormal proteins

    Vitamin K-dependent factors
    Factor VIII and von Willebrand factor
    Fibrinogen

Decreased clearance function

    Activated coagulation factors
    Plasminogen activators
    Thrombin-antithrombin III complexes

Abnormalities of platelets

    Disseminated intravascular coagulation
    Lipoproteins

From Lee CA, et al. Oxford Textbook of Clinical Hepatology. By permission of Oxford University Press, 1991.

Patients with chronic liver disease often have an associated vitamin K deficiency, either due to decreased absorption or because they are unable to utilize vitamin K due to hepatocellular dysfunction. Consequently, all vitamin K-dependent factors may be deficient in these patients. Although nonfunctional vitamin K precursors continue to be produced in these patients, they are not helpful in coagulation.[13]

Patients with chronic liver disease may have ongoing fibrinolysis due to increased levels of circulating plasminogen activators.[1,6,7,8,16] These levels are elevated due to decreased clearance and reduced inhibition of plasmin that result from the diminished synthesis of plasmin inhibitors in patients with chronic liver disease. When levels of circulating plasminogen activators are elevated prior to transplant, they obviously pose a significant problem during the transplant procedure.[19]

Disseminated intravascular coagulation, which may be subclinical, may also occur in patients with liver disease.[21,22] This condition may be caused by increased activation of clotting factors due to the release of thromboplastic material in the presence of a reduced concentration of the main inhibitory proteins. The presence of impaired removal of activated clotting factors and increased fibrinolytic activity may also contribute to this condition.

All of the above are common findings in the assessment of a patient about to undergo a liver transplant or in a patient with chronic liver disease about to undergo any surgical procedure. None of these findings provide a firm indication of a patient's true bleeding risk. I agree with earlier presenters that a history of prior bleeding problems is the best indication of the likelihood of bleeding problems during surgery. Among other indicators of bleeding risk (Table 3), prothrombin time (PT) may be a good indicator of liver status. Failure of PT to respond to vitamin K given parenterally may indicate significant hepatocellular dysfunction. Fibrinogen levels may fall as liver diseases worsen. Fibrin split products may provide the only indication of an ongoing lowgrade DIC. Bleeding time is not particularly helpful in the assessment of bleeding risk in patients with chronic liver disease.

Table 3. Indicators of Bleeding Risk in Patients With Liver Disease

Prothromin time

Platelet count

Fibrinogen level

Fibrin split products

Bleeding time

There are multiple approaches to the treatment of hemorrhage in liver disease (Table 4). A team approach is critical, with anesthesiologists and surgeons communicating and working closely together to monitor bleeding and to intervene with appropriate therapies. Often a very aggressive approach by both anesthesiologists and surgeons is required to maintain adequate hemostasis.

Table 4. Treatment of Hemorrhage in Liver Disease

Vitamin K

Fresh-frozen plasma

Cryoprecipitate

Platelet concentrates

Factor concentrates (rare)

1-Deamino-(8-D-arginine)-vasopressin

Aminocaproic acid

Aprotinin

The quality of the transplanted liver is vitally important to how well the patient clots in the intra- and perioperative periods, and good preservation of donor liver is essential. At the Texas Medical Center, we achieve very low intraoperative mortality rates when doing liver transplants, even with very sick patients, by precise surgical control of hemostasis, excellent anesthesia support, and replacement of a diseased liver with a well-functioning transplanted liver.

References

1. Bontempo FA, Lewis JH, Vanthiel DH, et al. The relation of preoperative coagulation findings to diagnosis, blood usage and survival in adult liver transplantation. *Transplantation* 1985;39:352.

2. Kang Y, Lewis JH, Navalgund A, Russell MW, Bontempa FA, Niren LS, Starzl TE. Epsilon-aminocaproic acid for treatment of fibrinolysis during liver transplantation. *Anesthesiology* 1987;66:766.

3. Kang YG, Martin DJ, Marquez J, et al. Intraoperative changes in blood coagulation and thrombelastographic monitoring in liver transplantation. *Anesth Analg* 1985;64:888.

4. Owen CA, Tettke SR, Bowie EJW, et al. Hemostatic evaluation of patients undergoing liver transplantation. *Mayo Clin Proc* 1987;62:761.

5. Palareti G, DeRosa V, Fortunato G, et al. Control of hemostasis during orthotopic liver transplantation. *Fibrinolysis* 2 1988;(suppl)3:61.

6. Porte RJ, Knot EAR. Haemostasis in liver transplantation. *Gastroenterology* 1989;97:488.

7. Carr JM. Hemostatic disorders in liver disease. In: Schiff L, Schiff ER, eds. *Diseases of the Liver* 7th ed. Philadelphia, PA: JB Lippincott; 1993:1061-1076.

8. Chopra S, Griffin PH. Laboratory tests and diagnostic procedures in evaluation of liver disease. *Am J Med* 1985;79:221.

9. Kelly DA, Tuddenham EGD. Haemostatic problems in liver disease. *Gut* 1986;27:339.

10. Lee CA, Kernoff PBA, Hutton RA. Effect of liver disease on other systems. haemostasis in liver disease. In: McIntyre N, Behanmou J, Bircher J, Rizzetto M, Rhodes J, eds. *Oxford Textbook of Clinial Hepatology.* vol. 2. Oxford: Oxford University Press; 1991:1234-1240.

11. Mannucci PM, Vicente V, Vianello L, et al. Controlled trial of desmopressin liver cirrhosis and other conditions associated with a prolonged bleeding time. *Blood* 1986;67:1148.

12. Stein SF, Harker LA. Kinetic and functional studies of platelets, fibrinogen, plasminogen in patients with hepatic cirrhosis. *J Lab Clin Med* 1982;99:217.

13. Boks A, Brommer EJP, Schalm SW, Van Vliet HHDM. Hemostasis and fibrinolysis in severe liver failure and their relation to hemorrhage. *Hepatology* 1986;6:79-86.

14. Dzik WH, Arkin CF, Jenkins RL, Stump DC. Fibrinolysis during liver transplantation in humans. role of tissue-type plasminogen activator. *Blood* 1988;71:1090.

15. Francis J, Armstrong DJ. Acquired dysfibrinogenemia in liver disease. *J Clin Pathol* 1982;35:667.

16. Francis RB Jr, Feinstein DI. Clinical significance of accelerated fibrinolysis in liver disease. *Haemostasis* 1984;14:460.

17. Martinez J, Keane PM, Gilman PB. The abnormal carbohydrate composition of the dysfibrinogenemia associated with liver disease. *Ann NY Acad Sci* 1983;408:388.

18. Sprengers ED, Kluft C. Plasminogen activator inhibitors. *Blood* 1987;69:381.

19. Knot E, Ten Cate JW, Drifhout HR, et al. Antithrombin III metabolism in patients with liver disease. *J Clin Pathol* 1984;37:523.

20. Kelly DA, O'Brien FJ, Hutton RA, et al. The effect of liver disease on factors V, VIII and protein C. *Br J Haematol* 1985;61:541.

21. Carr, JM. Disseminated intravascular coagulation in cirrhosis. *Hepatology* 1989;10:103.

22. Verstraete M, Vermylen J, Collen D. Intravascular coagulation in liver disease. *Annu Rev Med* 1974;25:447.

Clinical Significance
of Perioperative Bleeding
in Organ Transplantation

Valluvan Jeevanandam, MD

Bleeding after any procedure is problematic, but particularly so after organ transplantation. Transplantation frequently is done in patients with end-stage liver or cardiac disease; a good outcome in these very sick patients requires successful surgery and postoperative management, both of which are significantly complicated by bleeding.

Hemorrhagic death is the most obvious of the possible consequences of bleeding. Surgical technique may sometimes contribute to hemorrhagic death; for example, if a patient is closed while there is still residual bleeding from suture needle holes and hemostatic mechanisms subsequently fail to function, the patient may go into tamponade, form abscesses, or bleed out from the liver and require reexploration. Fortunately, the incidence of hemorrhagic death purely from bleeding is only about 0% to 3%, owing to the many surgical techniques available to salvage bleeding patients.

But bleeding requires transfusions, and transfusions come at a high price in both money and morbidity. First, the economic costs: Units of blood vary in cost from $100 to $300, depending on the region of the country; albumin, fresh-frozen plasma (FFP), and platelets all involve additional costs. Transfusions because of perioperative bleeding also involve a societal cost, depleting often scarce blood supplies and leaving less blood available for trauma or other cases in which hemostatic mechanisms cannot be controlled.

Patients who start to bleed tend to continue bleeding, since the bleeding itself increases fibrinolysis and procoagulant consumption. Because extended bleeding requires a large quantity of blood products, prevention of bleeding can dramatically decrease blood requirements.

Operative bleeding also clearly lengthens operating time, which is very costly in most institutions. To prevent the likelihood of having a patient return to the operating room to correct rebleeding, considerable time must be taken to ensure a dry field before closing the patient and sending him to the intensive care unit (ICU). This can consume 2 to 3 hours in a coagulopathic patient.

Extensive bleeding, defined as either rebleeding or bleeding requiring the transfusion of more than 5 units of red cells, significantly increases ICU and hospital stays. In a study of 120 heart transplant patients, among whom about 20 received aprotinin and the others did not, the average ICU stay was 3.2 days for patients with no bleeding and 7.1 days for patients with bleeding. The economic costs of operative bleeding thus clearly go far beyond just the costs of blood products.

Disease transmission is another serious consequence of transfusion. Although the transmission of hepatitis by transfusion is decreasing and now occurs with only about 1 of every 5,000 units of blood, the cases of hepatitis that do occur after organ transplantation with immunosuppression can be more virulent than those occurring in nonimmunosuppressed patients and are associated with greater morbidity and mortality. Furthermore, new viruses continue to be identified. We now know about hepatitis A, B, C, and D, but there may well be other types of hepatitis that we are not yet monitoring for. As was the case with the human immunodeficiency virus (HIV), a new virus may be identified in the future as causing syndrome X and only retrospectively will we discover that the virus may have been transmitted via transfusion. This raises the frightening possibility that transfusion transmission rates for still unknown diseases may be greater than the rates for the diseases we know about.

Cytomegalovirus (CMV) is a serious problem in organ transplantation, either when reactivated in a CMV-positive patient or when transmitted by transfusion. Although not a problematic illness in a normal population, CMV can cause serious gastritis or pneumonitis in an immunosuppressed transplant patient, which can be fatal. It also causes long-term effects in grafts, causing coronary artery disease in transplanted hearts and nephrosclerosis in transplanted kidneys. The treatment of CMV is expensive, requiring the intravenous administration of gancyclovir twice daily for 14 days. Patients sometimes require multiple hospital admissions. Moreover, CMV-negative blood is very scarce and difficult to obtain. Leukocyte-depleted blood is costly, and it still has not been proved that leukocyte depletion can prevent the transmission of CMV disease.

Complications in the wound and surgical incision area are another consequence of operative bleeding. Intra-abdominal bleeding may lead to the formation of seromas, which constitute an excellent culture medium, and intra-abdominal abscesses may develop. An intra-abdominal abscess in an immunosuppressed patient requires intensive treatment with antibiotics and may lead to graft loss. There is the possibility that antibiotics combined with cyclosporin may be nephrotoxic. In thoracic situations, bleeding is related to the incidence of sternal wound infection, which is associated with a 10% mortality in patients with heart transplants. Sternal wound infections obviously lengthen hospital stays and often require adjunct procedures.

Transfusions also alter the immune system. Studies have shown that blood transfusions during colorectal and hip procedures can increase the incidence of post-operative infections. There is also an increased rate of colon cancer recurrence in these patients. Mechanisms causing alterations of the immune system include formation of anti-idiotypic antibodies to FC fragments, increase in suppressor cell activity, down-regulation of the antigen-presenting cells, and a decrease in circulating lymphocytes. This can be advantageous after transplant surgery, as there can be a lower incidence of cellular rejection. With renal transplantation, donor-specific transfusion has been shown to decrease rejection and increase graph survival. However, excessive blood transfusions during a surgical procedure can increase the rate of infection and hence increase morbidity and mortality.

Sensitization can also occur with blood transfusions. Anti-HLA antibodies can be formed that cause accelerated acute rejection as well as chronic vascular rejection. These antibodies can be formed either through denovo synthesis or through an amnestic response. Formation of these antibodies is attenuated by leuckodepletion. Therefore, almost any patient who needs blood transfusions before or after transplantation should have pure leuckodepleted blood. Sensitization and the formation of accelerated or vascular rejection is very difficult to treat. Some forms of treatment include plasmapharesis, cytoxan since it has specific inhibitory capabilities for the B lymphocytes, and antibody-absorbing columns such as Prosorba.

Not only is the immune system altered after transfusion, but there is also an intrinsic inflammatory response. This has been documented by activation of elastase and interleukin-6 (IL-6) and interleukin-8 (IL-8) levels after excessive blood transfusions. Inflammatory-system activation can lead to adult respiratory distress syndrome (ARDS) and shocked lung, which in turn can lead to prolonged intubation, increased oxygen gradient and pulmonary vascular resistance, and incidence of right-side heart failure. In addition, a capillary leak syndrome can cause a patient to become edematous and retain volume.

All the above are consequences of bleeding and requirements for transfusion. How can bleeding be prevented? The number one cause of bleeding is surgical and this is prevented by correcting "suture deficiency" and exhaustive use of the electrocautery, especially in reoperations. Besides surgical bleeding, one needs to "correct the abnormal." In other words, preoperative thrombocytopenia and aspirin use can be corrected with platelets. Patients with congenital coagulation protein deficiencies can be corrected either with FFP or specific factor replacement. Many patients are anticoagulated preoperatively with warfarin and can be reversed with vitamin K. We have administered intravenous vitamin K while patients are in the operating room awaiting transplant. Patients remain hemodynamically stable and we are able to correct their prothrombin time in a matter of hours.[1] Uremia is a factor that can affect renal transplant patients, and these patients probably should be dialyzed before undergoing transplantation. Other measures to decrease bleeding include adjuncts to coagulation such as ε-aminocaproic acid (a fibrinolytic-suppressing agent) and aprotinin, a serum protease inhibitor that can suppress the inflammatory response as well as decrease bleeding.

Renal and pancreas transplants are not associated with generalized coagulopathy and excessive bleeding. Most bleeding in this situation would be surgical. The liver transplant surgeon faces a different task. Due to decrease synthesis of coagulant proteins, lack of fibrinolytic protein clearance, the use of veno bypass and an increase in tissue plasminogen activator levels, coagulopathy after liver transplantation is common. Patrassi et al reported an experimental double-blinded study of aprotinin in liver transplant patients and found a decrease by 50% in the number of blood products required and decreased length of operations.[2] Lung transplantation is particularly problematic with regard to bleeding: There is a lot of posterior mediastinal dissection, and bleeding with replacement therapy can lead to severe pulmonary dysfunction. This superimposed on ischemic lung injury can lead to primary donor failure. Aprotinin has been shown to decrease the fluid requirement and improve graft function after lung transplantation.[3,4]

With heart transplantation, there is an increased incidence of bleeding due to the preoperative coagulapathy state of the patients in addition to many anastomoses. We have used aprotinin in patients undergoing resternotomy for heart transplant and have shown that we can decrease blood product requirements by 75%.[5] There is also improvement in the first postoperative day alveolar-arterial oxygen gradient, with a subsequent decrease in time on the ventilator and in the ICU. There is a less positive fluid balance as well. We have given half-dose aprotinin with careful monitoring of renal function, especially in conjunction with patients getting cyclosporine. The one complication we have seen after aprotinin use is that immediate reexposure within a period of a month in some patients can cause anaphylactic reactions.

In conclusion, bleeding can cause a myriad of adverse effects in patients undergoing transplantation. Prevention is the best cure, with primary attention paid to surgical technique. Deficiencies in patients need to be corrected, and adjuncts to hemostasis such as aprotinin can be used in selected cases to decrease bleeding and improve function after transplantation.

References

1. Schweiger JW, Barnette RE, Brister NW, Weaver JP, Jeevanandam V. Rapid reversal of warfarin effect with intravenous vitamin K pre-cardiac transplant. *Crit Care Med* 1995;23:A6.

2. Patrassi GM, Viero M, Sartori MT, DeSilvestro G, Rossaro L, Burra P, Nolli ML, Piccinni P, Bassi N. Aprotinin efficacy on intraoperative bleeding and transfusion requirements in orthotopic liver transplantation. *Transfusion* 1994;34:507-511.

3. Jaquiss RD, Huddleston CB, Spray TL. Use of aprotinin in pediatric lung transplantation. *J Heart Lung Transplant* 1995;14:302-307.

4. Kesten S, de Hoyas A. Chapparo C, Westney G, Winton T, Maurer JR. Aprotinin reduces blood loss in lung transplant recipients. *Ann Thorac Surg* 1995:59:877-879.

5. Jeevanandam V, Furukawa S, Prendergast TP, Eisen HJ, McClurken JB. Defining the role of Aprotinin in orthotopic heart transplantation. Society of Thoracic Surgeons, Orlando 1996.

Reperfusion Physiology and Its Clinical Relevance

Keith A. A. Fox, MB, ChB, FRCP

Contractile changes are manifested at tissue, not cellular, level. Ischemic injury to myocardium is manifested in contractile, biochemical, and structural changes. Contractile changes occur due to systolic expansion and wall thinning; onset is within seconds of the initiation of ischemia. Biochemical changes include transient glycolytic flux, with onset at about 45 seconds of ischemia; hydrogen lactate accumulation; hydrolysis of high-energy phosphates; accumulation of intracellular calcium; and beta-oxidation inhibition. Structural changes may be either reversible or irreversible. Reversible changes occur within the first 20 minutes of zero flux; they include glycogen depletion, margination of nuclear chromatin, and myofibrillar edema. Irreversible changes occur at 40 to 60 minutes of zero flux; they include mitochondrial and sarcoplasmic swelling, deposit of lipid and protein in the mitochondria, and disruption of sarcolemma.

It is useful to distinguish between reperfusion phenomena, which occur on the reperfusion of already lethally injured myocardium, and true reperfusion injury that damages potentially viable myocardium. The latter is the subject of this review.

The most evident manifestations of reperfusion injury are arrhythmias, including premature ventricular beats, ventricular tachycardia, and ventricular fibrillation. Other injury manifestations include myocardial stunning; the accelerated expansion of necrosis; microvascular injury, with reflow either absent or impaired; myocardial hemorrhage; and lethal cell injury. Inflammatory responses are accelerated, with a series of inflammatory markers clearly implicated in reperfusion injury. These include cytokine pathways, neutrophil activation, and complement activation. Interestingly, the cytokine pathways that are affected in reperfusion injury to the heart are exactly the same as the pathways affected in acute lung injury and the adult respiratory distress syndrome (ARDS).

The no-reflow or impaired-reflow phenomenon that occurs in reperfusion injury has been demonstrated in experimental animal studies.[1] When an occlusion was induced within the left anterior descending artery, defects both in perfusion and extraction of a labeled fatty acid were quantified after reperfusion, using either microspheres or positron-labeled markers. Sequential tomography showed hyperemic reflow immediately on reperfusion in the myocardial zone previously ischemic due to the occlusion. Reperfusion within the first hour resulted in a very substantial return of perfusion. After 4 to 6 hours of ischemia, there was either no reflow or impaired reflow, with perfusion only 60% to 70% of the baseline level. This absence or impairment of reflow occurred in the presence of epicardial coronary arteries that were completely patent. Twenty-four hours later, both flow and fatty-acid extraction remained impaired, even though the involved vessels appeared totally patent on examination.[2]

Factors that affect the impact of both ischemia and reperfusion include the duration and severity of the ischemia, oxygen demand, collateral flow, stunning, hemorrhage, and tissue edema. The most critical factors in attempts to modify the impact of ischemia and reperfusion are limitation of the duration and severity of the ischemia and the staging of reflow to limit hyperemia. Other factors that can modify the impact of ischemia and reperfusion include hypothermia and cardioplegia, preconditioning, and the induction of stress proteins.

The abruptness of the return of reflow clearly affects the risk of ventricular fibrillation. After 20 minutes of ischemia in a cat model, the incidence of ventricular fibrillation was 60% to 65% with the abrupt return of reflow, but only about 20% with staged reflow.[3] The incidence of ventricular fibrillation after reperfusion clearly is also reduced by hypothermia and cardioplegia.

Murry et al[4] first studied the effect of repeated periods of ischemia on the myocardium. In a dog study, an experimental group was subjected first to four episodes of brief 5-minute periods of ischemia, with each ischemic period followed by reperfusion, and then to a prolonged period of 40 minutes of ischemia. The control group was simply subjected to the 40 minutes of ischemia, but no prior episodes (Fig l). The investigators expected myocardial injury to worsen with repeated episodes of ischemia. To their surprise, the infarct zone, expressed either in absolute terms or as a proportion of the area at risk, was reduced dramatically in the dogs preconditioned by the brief periods of ischemia. Infarct size was 7% of the ventricular area at risk in these animals compared with about 30% in the animals not previously subjected to the repeated brief periods of ischemia (Fig 2). This protective effect of preconditioning was subsequently demonstrated in repeated studies with other animal species.

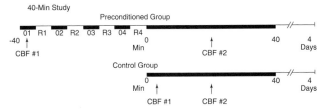

Fig 1. Preconditioning protocol: four periods of 5 minutes of circumflex coronary occlusion, each separated by 5 minutes of reperfusion (preconditioning group). Control and preconditioned animals then underwent 40 minutes of circumflex occlusion. Collateral blood flow (CBF) measured at points indicated; infarct size measured at 4 days of reperfusion. (Reproduced with permission from *Circulation.* 1986;74:1224-1126)

Fig 2. Infarct size and collateral blood flow (CBF) in animals with and without preconditioning (both subjected to 40 minutes of ischemia). Infarct size in control animals averaged 29.4% of area at risk and only 7.3% in preconditioned animals. Transmural mean collateral blood flow was not significantly different in the two groups. (Reproduced with permission from *Circulation.* 1986;74:1224-1126)

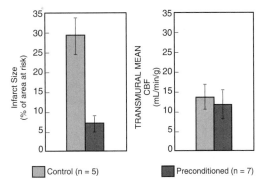

The salvage of myocardium that occurs with preconditioning cannot be attributed to the impact of collateral flow. In the absence of preconditioning, there is a semilinear relationship between collateral flow and infarct size, with infarct size increasing as collateral flow is reduced. But with preconditioning, numerous studies have shown that there is no clear relationship between collateral flow and infarct size. In the presence of preconditioning, infarct size as percentage of area at risk remains low over a wide range of collateral flow extending from very low to high.[4]

Preconditioning also decreases the rate of adenosine triphosphate (ATP) loss within the myocardium. Initially demonstrated in animal studies, preservation of myocardial ATP content also was shown in the first demonstration of preconditioning in the human myocardium. With the permission of their center's ethics committee, Yellon et al[5] subjected human hearts to pacing and crossclamp fibrillation as preconditioning prior to the prolonged ischemia of cardiopulmonary bypass (Fig 3). Needle biopsies of myocardial tissue were obtained before and after preconditioning and at the end of the first cross-clamp fibrillation.

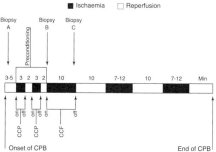

Fig 3. Preconditioning protocol in human hearts during cardiopulmonary bypass (CPB). Two episodes each of 3 minutes of crossclamp pacing (CCP) (90 beats/min). Needle biopsies were performed prior to preconditioning, immediately after preconditioning, and at the end of crossclamp fibrillation (ischemic interval). (Reproduced with permission from the Lancet Ltd. Yellon DM, Alkhulaifi AM, Pugsley WB. Preconditioning the human myocardium. *Lancet* 1993;342:276-277.)

In a control group without preconditioning, myocardial ATP content fell dramatically after the onset of ischemia. With preconditioning, although myocardial ATP content fell by the end of the preconditioning period, it then remained constant at that level throughout the period of ischemia, thus demonstrating preservation of tissue ATP content during the ischemic interval (Table 1).

Table 1. Adenosine Triphosphate Measurements in Preconditioned and Control Human Hearts.

	Before PC (biopsy A)	End of PC (biopsy B)	End of 1st CCF (biopsy C)
Group 1 (n = 7, PC)	20.6 (1.3)	10.5 (1.1)	12.0 (1.1)
Group 2 (n = 7, controls)	21.6 (1.6)	19.8 (1.3)	6.8 (0.2)

Results given as mean (SEM) in µmol/g dry weight. PC, preconditioning; CCF, crossclamp fibrillation. (Reproduced with permission from the Lancet Ltd. Yellon DM, Alkhulaifi AM, Pugsley WB. Preconditioning the human myocardium. *Lancet* 1993;342:276-277.)

In addition to reduction of infarct size and preservation of myocardial ATP content, preconditioning has been shown to reduce the frequency of reperfusion arrhythmias, reduce stunning, and preserve nerve function.[6] However, all the benefits of preconditioning wane if the period of ischemic insult is prolonged beyond 90 minutes and are totally lost if the ischemic interval lasts more than 3 hours. It should be noted, however, that there is evidence of a second window of protection that may last up to 24 hours.[7]

As for possible mechanisms involved in the cardioprotective effects of preconditioning, the use of specific antagonists to the adenosine-Al receptor has shown that this receptor is involved at least as part of the effector mechanism.[8] Preconditioning also causes activation of the potassium ATP channel and preconditioning has been shown to be blocked by inhibition of this channel with various antagonists.[9]

ATP-sensitive potassium channel openers (eg, cromokalim, nicorandil) are cardioprotective experimentally and may be used instead of ischemic preconditioning episodes to achieve [similar] cardioprotection. The action of these agents may be highly relevant to techniques of improving preservation. However, potassium ATP inhibitors (eg, glibenclamide) block preconditioning. There is evidence that this effect is mediated by a G protein that opens the potassium ATP channel.[10,11]

Thus, there are very exciting analogs available that may allow preconditioning. However, it must be noted that preconditioning of the heart requires normothermia; no one has yet been able to demonstrate preconditioning during hypothermia.

A family of myocardial stress proteins are synthesized in response to noxious stimuli. Inducing stimuli include raised temperature, the pressure of volume overload, some transition metals, free radicals, vasopressin, angiotensin, and isoproterenol. Myocardial stress proteins are not involved in preconditioning, which occurs too rapidly for transcriptional changes to take place, but represent a second mechanism of myocardial protection. The synthesis of these proteins results in an elevation of endogenous catalase, ATP preservation, and reduction of infarct size.[12] Stress proteins are not induced if ischemia is severe and prolonged.

The mechanisms reviewed above suggest that the future may hold exciting possibilities for improving myocardial preservation by use of agonists and antagonists of these mechanisms.

References

1.   Kloner RA, Przyklenk K. Consequences of ischemia. Reperfusion on the coronary microvasculature. In: Yellon DM, Jennings RB, eds. *The Pathophysiology of Reperfusion and Reperfusion Injury.* New York:Raven Press Ltd; 1992:85-104.

2.   Knabb RM, Bergmann SR, Fox KAA, Sobel BE. The temporal pattern of recovery of myocardial perfusion and metabolism delineated by positron emission tomography after coronary thrombolysis. *J Nucl Med* 1987;28(8): 1563-1570.

3.   Hearse DJ, Bolli R. Reperfusion-induced injury: manifestations, mechanisms, and clinical relevance. *Cardiovasc Res* 1992;26:101-108.

4.   Murry CE, Jennings RB, Reimer KA. Preconditioning with ischemia; a delay of lethal cell injury in ischemic myocardium. *Circulation* 1986;74:1124-1126.

5. Yellon DM, Alkhulaifi AM, Pugsley WB. Preconditioning the human myocardium. *Lancet* 1993;342:276-277.

6. Walker DM, Yellon DM. Ischaemic preconditioning: from mechanisms to exploitation. *Cardiovasc Res* 1992;26:734-739.

7. Marber MS, Latchman DS, Walker JM, Yellon DM. Cardiac stress protein elevation 24 hours after brief ischemia or heart stress is associated with resistance to myocardial infarction. *Circulation* 1993;88:1264-1272.

8. Liu GS, Thornton J, Van Winkle DM, Stanley AWH, Olsson KA, Downey JM. Protection against infarction afforded by preconditioning is mediated by A1 adenosine receptors in rabbit heart. *Circulation* 1991;84:350-356.

9. Sanguinetti MC, Scott AL, Zingaro GJ, Siegl PKS. BRL 34915 (cromakalim) activates ATP-sensitive K+ current in cardiac muscle. *Proc Natl Acad Sci USDAA* 1988;85:8360-8364.

10. Grover GJ. Protective effects of ATP-sensitive potassium channel openers in models of myocardial ischaemia. *Cardiovasc Res* 1994;28:778-782.

11. Hearse DJ. Activation of ATP-sensitive potassium channels: a novel pharmaco-logical approach to myocardial protection? *Cardiovasc Res* 1995;30:1-7.

12. Yellon DM, Latchman DS. Stress proteins and myocardial protection during ischaemia and reperfusion. In: Yellon DM, Jennings RB, eds. *The Pathophysiology of Reperfusion and Reperfusion Injury*. New York:Raven Press Ltd; 1992:185-194.

Long-Term Preservation in Organ Transplantation

Anthony M. D'Alessandro, MD

James H. Southard, PhD

The three major advances in organ transplantation in recent decades have been development of organ-preservation techniques, improved surgical techniques, and new immunosuppressive strategies. Organ preservation is closely linked to the challenge of hemostasis in organ transplantation, for without a well-preserved organ, hemostatic difficulties increase.

The first major advance in organ preservation occurred in 1967 when Belzer and Hoffmann developed a pulsatile, or machine perfusion technique capable of preserving kidneys for up to 72 hours.[1] In 1969, Collins introduced a much simpler method for kidney preservation, a solution that permitted cold storage of kidneys for up to 30 hours.[2] Belzer's machine perfusion and Collins solution remained the primary clinical methods available for organ preservation throughout most of the 1980s.

MACHINE ORGAN PRESERVATION

Our institution currently uses machine preservation of kidneys, clearly necessary because we transplant over 200 cadaveric kidneys annually. The increased safe preservation time of machine perfusion permits us to preserve many kidneys simultaneously and affords us the opportunity to perform kidney transplants during daytime hours, obviously a welcome benefit for our surgeons, anesthesiologists, nurses, and other hospital personnel.

In 1989, successful 5-day preservation of the canine kidney by machine perfusion was achieved by adding 0.5 mM of calcium to the preservation solution and donor pretreatment with 2.5 mg/kg of chlorpromazine.[3] Preservation was not successful if calcium was either left out of the solution or provided in higher concentrations. In the absence of chlorpromazine, only 60% of kidneys survived for 5 days. Seven-day preservation of dog kidneys subsequently was achieved with the addition to the perfusion solution of furegrelate, a thromboxane A_2 (TxA_2) synthetase inhibitor.[4] However, the addition of aspirin, which blocks cyclooxygenase somewhat more proximally in the arachidonic acid cycle, resulted in no kidney survival. Thus, it appears necessary to maintain the prostacycline limb of the arachidonic acid while blocking TxA_2 to achieve 7-day perfusion preservation of the kidney.

Although 5- or 7-day organ preservation is not used clinically, better long-term preservation correlates directly with better short-term preservation, with important consequences for immediate function in the transplanted organs. Immediate function is obtained in 95% of transplanted kidneys at centers (University of Wisconsin, University of Alabama, Ohio State University) currently using machine preservation; this compares with the immediate function of 78% of transplanted kidneys preserved with cold storage in University of Wisconsin solution (Table l).[5-7]

Table 1. Perfusion Preservation in Human Kidney Transplantation

Type of preservation	Wisconsin UW-Perf	Alabama UW-Perf	Ohio State UW-Perf	Eurotransplant UW-Cold storage
Preservation time (h)	28 ± 8	29 ± 9	20 ± 5	24 ± 8
Kidneys (n)	183	188	140	352
Immediate function	95%	95%	98%	78%

UW, University of Wisconsin.

The need for dialysis after kidney transplant is directly related to the cold ischemic time of the transplanted kidney, ranging from 20% with kidneys preserved with cold ischemic times of 1 to 12 hours to 37% with kidneys preserved for over 48 hours (Table 2). Additionally, it is becoming apparent that long-term graft survival is about 10% better when transplanted kidneys function well immediately than when they do not (Fig 1).

Table 2. Dialysis and Cold Ischemic Time

Cold Ischemic Time (h)	Kidneys (n)	Dialysis (%)
1 to 5	652	20
6 to 12	1876	20
13 to 24	5812	22
25 to 48	6014	33
> 48	508	37
Total	**14,862**	**26**

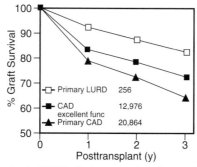

Fig 1. Overall graft survival. LURD, living unrelated renal donation; CAD, cadaveric. (Reprinted with permission from Clinical Transplants 1994, UCLA Tissue Typing Laboratory.)

COLD-STORAGE ORGAN PRESERVATION

With the advent of cyclosporine in 1983, extrarenal transplant programs blossomed. However, existing methods that permitted preservation of kidneys for up to 30 hours or more proved inadequate for the liver or the pancreas, which could be preserved for only 6 hours. Belzer then undertook a research program to develop a cold-storage solution that would meet the clinical need for preservation of a pancreas for up to 30 hours and a liver for up to 18 hours. What has become known as the UW (University of Wisconsin) solution was the outcome of this program.

Organ preservation is a multifactorial phenomenon, with prominent roles played by temperature, solution, and reperfusion effects, among other factors. Storage of the organ at hypothermia obviously is essential; if the organ's warm ischemic tolerance is assumed to be 1 hour, it can be increased to 13 hours simply by using cold heparinized blood. Using an appropriate solution in conjunction with hypothermia further extends preservation of the organ up to 48 hours or more in the case of the kidney. The solution has effects on both the physical and biochemical environments of the organ being preserved.

Solution Effects on Physical Environment of Organs

Factors to be considered in the organ's physical environment include osmotic factors, electrolytes, buffer solutions, and colloids. Osmotic factors are controlled by using impermeants, which keep cells from swelling during hypothermic storage. We currently use the anion lactobionate for this purpose in our cold-storage solution and gluconate as the major anion in our machine perfusion. Basically, both substances prevent cell swelling by replacing chloride, a permeable anion, which takes water into cells in organs that are hypothermically preserved.

Tissue studies showed that a variety of saccharides are also important to prevent cell swelling. Glucose is the major impermeant in Collins solution, but, as a relatively small molecule, it enters cells and is metabolized. Raffinose is the major saccharide contained in the UW solution; as a large molecule, it has proved very effective in preventing cell swelling.

The major colloid contained in the UW solution is hydroxyethyl starch. Although the need for such a colloid in a cold-storage preservation solution has been questioned, we believe that it provides a better flush-out of the organ when it is removed.

Solution Effects on Biochemical Environment of Organs

With respect to solution effects on the biochemical environment of preserved organs, we found that the addition of adenosine to the preservation solution greatly increased adenosine triphosphate (ATP) regeneration and decreased lactate dehydrogenase (LDH) release, a measure of cell damage, in renal tubules that were stored for 48 hours (Fig 2).

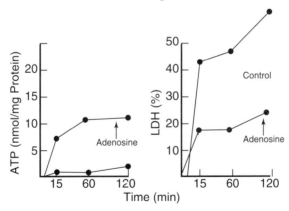

Fig 2. Effect of adenosine on kidneys cold-stored for 48 hours. ATP, adenosine triphosphate; LDH, lactate dehydrogenase.

Clearly, adenosine plus phosphate promotes ATP regeneration during cold-storage preservation. Although we do not use adenosine in our machine perfusate, we do include adenine and ribose, which give better long-term ATP regeneration at 5 and 7 days. Glutathione is an oxygen-free radical scavenger that also acts to protect sulfhydryl containing proteins. We found that glutathione, like adenosine, also promotes ATP regeneration and reduces LDH release in stored renal tubules (Fig 3). Since glutathione breaks down quite rapidly once it is added to the preservation solution, we currently add it to the UW solution just before leaving for an organ retrieval.

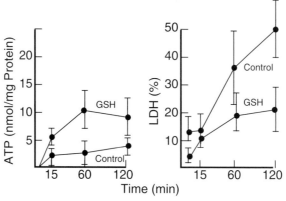

Fig 3. Effect of glutathione on kidney cells cold-stored for 48 hours. ATP, adenosine triphosphate; LDH, lactate dehydrogenase; GSH, glutathione.

When the UW cold-storage solution was developed, using these studies as guides to the selection of its final composition, its effectiveness was first studied in a series of experimental pancreas transplants. Wahlberg et al achieved 3-day preservation of the pancreas in a canine model with the solution.[8] Jamieson et al achieved 48-hour preservation of the canine liver, which never before had been accomplished.[9]

The major components of the UW solution that have been experimentally shown to play important roles in organ preservation are lactobionic acid, glutathione, adenosine, raffinose, and hydroxyethyl starch. The importance of some of the minor components of the solution, such as dexamethasone, allopurinol, magnesium, antibiotics, and insulin, has not been experimentally established. However, these components were parts of the solution as originally developed and have been retained, because of suggestive evidence of their efficacy in suppression preservation injury.

Cold-Stored Pancreas-Renal Transplants

An early clinical series of 253 cases of combined pancreas and renal transplants using organs cold-stored with the UW solution showed only one patient who was not immediately insulin-independent and one case of primary nonfunction, two of vascular thrombosis, and one of graft pancreatitis. Hemodialysis was required after transplantation in only 2.4% of cases.

In this series, kidneys were stored for about 18 hours and pancreases for about 17 hours. None of the pancreas transplants were done at night; all were done the morning after procurement. We have continued with this scheduling practice because the positive results obtained clearly showed that more prompt transplantation was not required.

In a somewhat later series of 277 combined pancreas and renal transplants, various parameters of pancreatic and renal function were measured. The mean fasting blood glucose was within normal range at day l, day 7, and at discharge. The mean serum amylase, which together with the urine amylase provides an indication of exocrine preservation, was 322 IU on day l. Levels of urinary amylase rose sharply and levels of creatinine fell sharply from day l to day 7 and then to discharge.

The record of long-term organ survival with the UW solution also suggests that the solution is clinically adequate for pancreas and kidney preservation. In the series of 253 combined pancreas-renal transplants, kidney survival was 89% at 1 year and 80% at 5 years. Pancreas survival was 86% at 1 year and 78% at 5 years.

Cold-Stored Liver Transplants

Subsequent to our very early clinical experience with preservation of the pancreas with UW solution, we used it to preserve the liver. The first human semielective liver transplant was performed at the University of Wisconsin Hospital in August 1987. The liver was stored for 2l hours and functioned well immediately after transplantation. Based on this early experience, we began to preserve livers in UW solution overnight and not perform liver transplants at night. Thus, prior to 1993, the mean preservation time of the livers we transplanted was close to 13 hours. However, our experience of a somewhat increased rate of nonfunction or poor function when preservation times approached 16 to 17 hours led us to reverse our policy and to again begin performing the transplants immediately, day or night.[10] Our mean preservation time then went down to about 10 hours.

With overnight liver preservation and the longer mean preservation time, we had a 6% nonfunction rate and a 16% rate of initial poor function in 391 transplants. Since reverting to immediate transplantation, and with the introduction of a biopsy protocol in which we histologically examine the liver, we have had only two cases of nonfunction and an 11% rate of initial poor function in 160 transplants.

OTHER INFLUENCES ON TRANSPLANTED ORGANS

Factors other than preservation method and time influence the functioning of transplanted organs. Various donor and recipient factors have an important role, particularly in a procedure as complex as liver transplantation. A multivariate analysis showed that steatosis in the donor liver, reduction or splitting of the liver, older donor age, recipient retransplantation, and recipient renal insufficiency all influence outcomes, as does longer cold-storage times (Table 3).[10]

Table 3. Effect of Risk Factors on Multivariate Analysis of Liver Transplantaton	
Factor	**IF-IPF-PNF**
Fatty donor liver biopsy	0.006
Reduced liver	0.001
Older donor age	0.009
Retransplantation	0.01
Renal insufficiency	0.02
Longer cold storage	0.02

IF, Initial function; IPF, initial poor function; PNF, primary nonfunction.

PRESENT AND FUTURE BENEFITS

The successful introduction of the UW solution spurred increased interest in organ-preservation research. The solution's action in increasing preservation time for most organs permitted the utilization of more organs, which now may be procured at greater distance. Surgery can be performed electively, and a hospital thus needs only a single transplant team. Increasing the likelihood of early organ functioning may contribute to significantly reduced hospital costs.

The factors that affect safe organ preservation — (namely, ischemia, hypothermia, solution, biochemical, and perfusion) — have an additive effect. Developing preservation methods based on understanding each factor increases the length of time that organs can be preserved experimentally (Table 4). Our research efforts have now come full circle, with renewed attention being given to perfusion effects on organ preservation. It may be that the truly long-term pulsatile preservation achieved with kidneys may also be feasible for livers. More than a decade of laboratory efforts led us to design and construct a pulsatile perfusion machine that will accommodate a liver, with possible application to other organs.

Table 4. Factors Important in Organ Preservation				
Factor	**Kidney**	**Liver**	**Pancreas**	**Heart**
Ischemia (37° C)	1 h	1 h	30 min	15-30 min
Hypothermia (4°C)	12 h	2-3 h	?	1-2 h
Solution effect	30-48 h	6-10 h	6-10 h	4-6 h
Biochemical effect	72 h	48 h	72 h	12-24 h
Perfusion effect	120 h	72 h	96 h	24-48 h

The future of organ preservation will surely see the development of better short-term preservation solutions for all organs and better long-term preservation of some organs. Attention is now being focused on methods to salvage organs from less than ideal donors, such as nonheart-beating donors; there is some experimental evidence that the effects of warm ischemia can be mitigated with perfusion preservation. In the future, we may learn to immunologically alter organs during preservation. Eventually, we may learn to successfully cryopreserve organs for truly long-term storage.

References

1. Belzer FO, Ashby BS, Dunphy JE. 24- and 72-hour preservation of canine kidneys. *Lancet* 1967;2:536-538.

2. Collins GM, Bravo-Shugarman M, Terasaki PI. Kidney preservation for transplantation: initial perfusion and 30-hour ice storage. *Lancet* 1969;2:1219-1222.

3. McAnulty JF, Ploeg RJ, Southard JH, et al. Successful five-day perfusion preservation of the canine kidney. *Transplantation* 1989;47:37-41.

4. Schilling M, Saunder A, Southard JH, et al. Five- to seven-day kidney preservation with aspirin and furegrelate. *Transplantation* 1993;55:955-958.

5. Barber WH, Hudson SL, Deierhoi MH, et al. Pulsatile perfusion preservation: early posttransplant dialysis requirement predicts rapid graft loss. *Transplant Proc* 1990;22:446-447.

6. Henry ML, Sommer BG, Tesi RJ, et al. Improved immediate renal allograft function after initial simple cold storage. *Transplant Proc* 1990;22:388-389.

7. Ploeg RJ, Hajo van Bockel J, Langendijk PTH, et al. Effect of preservation solution on results of cadaveric kidney transplantation. *Lancet* 1992;340:129-137.

8. Wahlberg JA, Love R, Landegaard L, Southard JH, Belzer FO. 72-hour preservation of the canine pancreas. *Transplantation* 1987;43:5-8.

9. Jamieson NV, Sundberg R, Lindell S, et al. Preservation of the canine liver for 24 to 48 hours using simple cold storage with UW solution. *Transplantation* 1988;46:517-522.

10. Ploeg RJ, D'Alessandro AM, Knechtle SJ, et al. Risk factors for primary dysfunction after liver transplantation: a multivariate analysis. *Transplantation* 1993;55:807-813.

Hemostatic Difficulties in Liver Transplantation

Robert A. Fisher, MD

The great variability seen in studies seeking to identify factors associated with morbidity and mortality in liver transplantation is a reflection of the procedure's attendant complexities. These include variability in surgical reconstruction; level of liver dysfunction of individual patients in a study; and effects on the physiology of hemostasis of mechanical factors or operative procedures. Analysis is further complicated by the extent to which hemostatic difficulty encountered is attributable to existing decompensation of the patient's liver. The degree of preexisting immunosuppression in a patient with chronic cirrhosis before drug administration and of technical difficulties related to number of previous abdominal procedures; extent of ascites; degree of thrombocytopenia due to splenic enlargement; and the presence of kidney tubular dysfunction or hidden clot are all unquantitated variables of survival (Fig 1).[1]

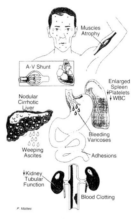

Fig 1. Preexisting factors prior to transplantation that may influence perioperative hemostatic management.

In liver transplantation, the experience of the transplant team is one factor that appears undeniably related both to the amount of blood loss and to technical satisfaction of the operative procedure. Four studies reported by highly experienced transplant teams that involved 755 adult and 238 pediatric liver transplant procedures clearly show that the blood requirement of both adult and pediatric patients had no correlation with any specific preoperative coagulation test or any combination of such tests.[2-5] Deakin[3] and Mor[4] found that the presence of renal dysfunction measured either by creatinine or by blood urea nitrogen (BUN), as well as thrombocytopenia and the presence of a patient in the hospital or in the intensive care unit (ICU) prior to liver transplantation, were associated with increased blood-product use during the transplant procedure. In addition, these two studies and the one from Gerlach and associates[5] show a strong correlation between perioperative transfusion rates and postoperative infections and mortality. Patients hospitalized prior to their transplant procedure because of failing livers or related complications had the worst outcomes. These findings underscore the need to critically evaluate the preoperative condition of patients, including overall nutritional depletion, when reviewing data on infection and morbidity in liver transplantation.

This presentation will address the coagulation disorders and difficulties in hemostasis associated with the three stages of liver transplantation: the recipient hepatectomy, the anhepatic stage, and postreperfusion to the time of closure.

Stage l: Recipient Hepatectomy

An enduring myth holds that patients with portal hypertension and bleeding, whether or not they have undergone a previous corrective procedure, are at increased risk of poor outcomes after transplantation. A 1993 review of patients with (n=70) and without (n=116) a variceal bleed prior to transplantation showed no correlation between this factor and posttransplant morbidity or survival.[6] Prior sclerotherapy or placement of a transjugular intrahepatic portacaval shunt (TIPS) or surgical shunt did not affect posttransplant outcome. The data suggest that we discard prior bleeding as a factor in the analysis of posttransplant outcomes.

Recent studies show that although blood loss is greater in patients who have had a prior portosystemic shunt, about twice that of patients without a prior shunt and averaging 27 units, the greater blood loss does not increase mortality in the presence of an experienced transplant team.[7,8] Many initially had hoped that TIPS might be done prophylactically to decrease blood loss in the operating room and possibly improve posttransplant outcomes. A recent review by Menegaux[9] noted that, although TIPS patients show less bleeding than patients treated with portacaval shunts, TIPS does not improve survival at 2 years. Somberg's[10] review of the NIDDK (National Institute of Diabetes and Digestive and Kidney Diseases) liver transplantation patient database compared operative outcomes of 41 patients with TIPS placed prior to transplant with results of 82 patients who had neither TIPS nor a portosystemic shunt to control portal hypertension before transplantation. There was absolutely no difference between the two groups in either operative blood loss or survival. Furthermore, additional complications that were factored out in the above study may occur when doing liver transplants in patients who have had prior TIPS. In our early experience with 15 TIPS patients at the time of liver transplantation, 2 patients developed fresh portal mesenteric thrombosis secondary to TIPS; and extension of the razor-edged metal conduits into the atrium and portal splenic vein junction in 2 patients led to increased operative blood loss and operative time and to the wounding of the surgeon, introducing the risk of hepatitis to the operator.

Metabolic problems encountered during the recipient hepatectomy stage include dilution, uremia, and imbalances of sodium and osmolality that represent a single group of variables in a complex setting of an open abdomen, as illustrated in Fig 2.

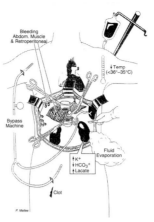

Fig 2. Mechanical and physiologic events during the operative procedure that may result in hemostatic difficulties.

In the last 235 liver transplants done under my direction, we commonly have used plasmapheresis in the preanhepatic stage, as described in l989 by Munoz,[11] attempting to improve patient coagulation profiles. We have used this procedure particularly in decompensated Child's C cirrhotic patients who were bleeding and stabilized with TIPS (n = 30) and in all patients prior to cerebral pressure monitor placement. The TIPS procedure increased patient survival time in the hospital to 90%, thus extending time to find a donor liver. Two- to- three-liter apheresis with fresh-frozen plasma (FFP) and cryoprecipitate replacement prevented the hemodynamic compromise of transferring pressure volume directly from the right side of the heart to the varices via the TIPS, at the same time providing clotting factors without dilution of hematocrit.

It has also become our standard practice in patients with either hepatorenal or acute renal failure, two conditions that are often indistinguishable, to intraoperatively dialyze these patients with a separate catheter in their internal jugular vein on the side opposite the rapid-infusion device. Heparin is not used for dialysis and is not used in the veno-veno bypass circuit.

Another standard practice in inhospital hyponatremic or ICU United Network of Organ Sharing (UNOS) status 1 patients is to maintain the patient's sodium and osmolality in a < 10 mEq/mosmol range by using tromethamine (THAM) buffer (rather than $NaHCO_3$) at the time of anesthetic induction. With this approach, the rare but devastating complications of pontine and extrapontine myelinolysis reported in these high-risk groups have not occurred.[12]

We also commonly use the inferior mesenteric vein as the portal segment for veno-veno bypass, as illustrated in Fig 2. This enables us to do a mass enclampment of the porta in patients with a very adherent porta, since we are able to get decompression through the inferior mesenteric system routinely with a 16-french William Harvey catheter (Fig 3). Even in the most difficult patients, I always attempt to leave the infrahepatic cava intact so as not to disturb the retroperitoneal varices. With the liver out of the way, it is much easier to deal with bleeding from the retroperitoneal and diaphragmatic bare areas and occasionally the adrenal orifice. At this juncture, cuff construction for "piggyback" or retrohepatic caval replacement can be decided for implantation of the liver.

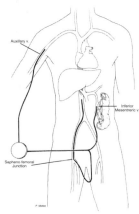

Fig 3. Use of a 16-gauge William Harvey catheter to achieve portal decompression through the inferior mesenteric system.

In six patients with platelet counts of less than 40,000/µL and symptomatic hypersplenism or incidental splenic artery aneurysm, I have ligated the splenic artery at its celiac junction without splenectomy. No splenic infarct or pancreatitis has occurred in these patients. Also, they did not require repeated platelet transfusions in the perioperative period, as is often the case in patients who are extremely hypersplenic and thrombocytopenic.

Extensive experience with segmental liver transplant has taught me the value of 3.5 loop magnification at the back table. This adjunct reduces the time needed to prepare the liver segments from 3 to 4 hours to 2 hours, without increasing blood loss from the raw surface of the segments. When placing segments, I have long added cryoprecipitate to raise the factor VIII level to 100%, especially in our adult patients. This ensures the availability of von Willebrand factor on reperfusion to help with platelet adhesion at the cut surface. This is followed by fibrin gluing of the surface, which appears to decrease the rate of seroma formation on the surface and may also be bactericidal. I also routinely use the argon beam coagulator to beam the segment capsule and the raw surface where I resect the caudate to prevent impingement on the portal vein. This impingement is a factor in thrombosis, especially when using a 9:1 segmental difference in a very small child.

For patient thermoregulation, the Omnitherm Heat Exchanger (Scimed Life Systems, Minneapolis, Minn) is used on the rapid infusion device (RID) and veno-veno bypass circuit, based on our prospective controlled study results of 20 consecutive liver transplant patients in whom we used the heat exchanger and 20 in whom we did not. Measurement by esophageal and rectal probe of changes in temperature in these patients documented that using the exchanger raised temperatures by an average of 2.1°C, with most patients having a body temperature of 36° to 37°C at termination of veno-veno bypass. Patients who did not have the heat exchanger generally showed a drop in temperature of 3 degrees. The difference was significant ($P=.001$) enough to justify routine use of the heat exchanger. We place the exchanger 3 feet from the patient's axillary input line and have not encountered any problems with thrombosis or hemolysis.

Stage 2: The Anhepatic Stage
Up to 40% of patients will show fibrinolysis during the anhepatic stage of liv-

er transplantation.[13,14] The mechanisms involved are well known: prothrombin time (PT), partial thromoplastin time (PTT), and activated PTT (aPTT) become elevated and in turn levels of tissue plasminogen activator (t-PA) increase. Further depletion of factors I, V, VII, and VIII follows, together with further depletion of platelets, calcium, and magnesium.

We administer magnesium at time of incision, especially in chronically debilitated patients. Correction of low magnesium and calcium serum levels has been shown to reduce catecholamine requirement in stress-induced myocardial depression.[15]

Liver transplantation is performed with an anesthesia team experienced in the use of thromboelastography. We thus obtain information at the operative table that otherwise might be very difficult to obtain promptly from the hemostasis laboratory, especially on holidays, weekends, and in the middle of the night. A recently published article elegantly reviews the thromboelastogram (TEG) information relevant to transplant procedures.[14] The uses to which I put the information gained from a TEG include using the factor-dependent reaction time to distinguish between a normal patient, a patient with factor deficiency, and a patient who has not had adequate replacement of FFP; this can be particularly important in a hemophiliac patient. The TEG also provides a simple estimation of the coagulation time, which is highly dependent on platelets. Therefore, when confronted with intraoperative muscle bleeding, the TEG profile may quickly show that there is a need for more platelets, before a platelet count has been returned from the laboratory. The TEG also may show that more platelets are needed even when a laboratory platelet count shows 80,000/mL, indicating that the platelets are insufficiently functional as is illustrated in Fig 4. And, of course, a rapid drop in maximum amplitude on the TEG indicates the presence of fibrinolysis.

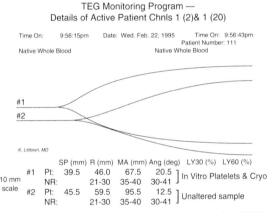

TEG Monitoring Program —
Details of Active Patient Chnls 1 (2)& 1 (20)

Time On: 9:56:15pm   Date: Wed. Feb. 22, 1995   Time On: 9:56:43pm
Patient Number: 111

Native Whole Blood   Native Whole Blood

#1
#2

K. Littlown, MD

		SP (mm)	R (mm)	MA (mm)	Ang (deg)	LY30 (%)	LY60 (%)	
#1	Pt:	39.5	46.0	67.5	20.5			] In Vitro Platelets & Cryo
10 mm scale	NR:		21-30	35-40	30-41			
#2	Pt:	45.5	59.5	95.5	12.5			] Unaltered sample
	NR:		21-30	35-40	30-41			

Fig 4. Effect of platelet and cryoprecipitate transfusion on the TEG profile. Blood was sampled from a patient before (trace 2) and after transfusion (trace 1). The profiles show transfusion improved clot formation with a decreased reaction (R) time, indicating a faster initiation of clot formation and an increase in the maximum amplitude (MA) of the trace reflecting improved clot strength.

Stage 3: Postreperfusion

The problems of the postreperfusion period are illustrated in the cartoon (Fig 5). These include temperature regulation; the possibility of an elevation of aPTT from a graft heparin effect, which can occur in 30% to 40% of patients; renal failure; and, rarely, the immunologic rejection of the liver, causing primary nonfunction and sometimes explosive fibrinolysis, described as a toxic liver syndrome. When the liver is nonfunctional, all the problems of hemostasis encountered in stage 2 are confounded.

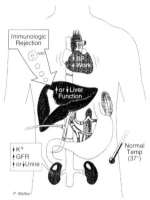

Fig 5. Potential problems associated with the postreperfusion period. GFR, Glomerular filtration rate.

Experience With Epsilon-Aminocaproic Acid

In 1987, the efficacy of low-dose ε-aminocaproic acid (EACA) in preventing severe fibrinolysis in liver transplantation without the risk of thrombosis seen with the higher dose was reported.[16] To gain confidence in using a lower-dose EACA in the most critical liver transplant patients, we prospectively evaluated administering 1 gram at incision followed by 250 mg/h until cross-clamping the liver vasculature and the start of bypass. The study involved six UNOS status 1 adult patients, all with liver failure and multiorgan failure and expected to die within 7 days. Randomly, three patients received EACA and three patients did not. Two of the patients had renal failure and required intraoperative dialysis. Two patients had active variceal bleeding entering the operative theater. Patients were matched for age, height, and weight and all were plasmapheresed before being brought to the operating room. Patient initial PTs remained high even after plasmapheresis (Table 1). Fibrinogen levels were corrected in control and treated groups due to the cryoprecipitate used in the plasmapheresis (Table 1). Levels of factor VII were partially improved by the administered volume of FFP prior to incision in both groups, although factor VII deficiency can never be completely corrected in patients with total liver failure (Table 1).

Table 1. Preoperative Coagulation Data forIndividual Study Patients

	Control			EACA		
	P 1	P 2	P 3	P 1	P 2	P 3
PT (sec)	15	24	15	23	21	22
Fibrinogen (mg/dL)	170	160	310	225	225	155
Factor VII (%)	24	16	44	13	24	21

EACA, ε-Aminocaproic acid; PT, prothrombin time.

Operative time was similar in both groups of patients through all three stages of the liver transplant procedure. Analysis of levels of factors V, VII, and VIII showed little difference between the two groups in stage 1, indicating that the anesthesia teams had competently performed the task of replacement. In stage 2, patients who received EACA showed no evidence of fibrinolysis and maintained greater than 100% factor VIII activity. The largest difference occurred in levels of factor VIII. Fibrinolysis that consumed factor VIII in the control patients may account for this difference. There was no difference between the two groups in factors V, VII, and VIII in stage 3 at the time of closure (Table 2).

Table 2. Coagulation Factor Levels and Surgical Operative Time for Each Stage of Liver Transplantation

| | Stage 1 | | Stage 2 | | Stage 3 | |
	Control	EACA	Control	EACA	Control	EACA
Factor V (%)	45	40	38	40	25	35
Factor VII (%)	30	25	40	37	40	50
Factor VIII (%)	195	175	70	130	100	105
Surgical time (min)	380	295	50	50	220	215

EACA, ε-Aminocaproic acid.

Analysis of blood use, including packed red blood cells (PRBCs), FFP, and platelets, showed no difference between the two groups in stage 1 and stage 3. Blood utilization was lower in the patients receiving EACA during stage 2 (Table 3). Thus, this study suggests that using EACA in a selected group of high-risk liver transplant patients *does* make a difference in blood utilization, similar to the conclusion reached in other studies.[16,17] These data also indicate that it is in stage 2, the stage in which we would anticipate that fibrinolysis would be most significant, that drug intervention makes a difference.

Table 3. Blood-Product Use for Each Stage of Liver Transplantation

| | Stage 1 | | Stage 2 | | Stage 3 | |
	Control	EACA	Control	EACA	Control	EACA
PRBCs (U)	7	5	5	2	4	7
FFP (U)	10	9	6	3	5	8
PLT (U)	20	17	5	3	20	19

EACA, ε-Aminocaproic acid; PRBCs, packed red blood cells; FFP, fresh-frozen plasma; PLT, platelets.

References:

1. Porte RJ. Coagulation and fibrinolysis in orthotopic liver transplantation. *Semin Thromb Hemost* 1993;19(3):191-196.

2. Carlier M, Van-Obbergh LJ, Veyckemans F, et al. Hemostasis in children undergoing liver transplantation. *Semin Thromb Hemost* 1993;19(3):218-222.

3. Deakin M, Gunson BK, Dunn JA, et al. Factors influencing blood transfusion during adult liver transplantation. *Ann Royal Coll Surg* 1993;75(5):339-344.

4. Mor E, Jennings L, Gonwa TA, et al. The impact of operative bleeding on outcome in transplantation of the liver. *Surg Gynecol Obstet* 1993;176:219-227.

5. Gerlach H, Slama KJ, Bechstein WO, et al. Retrospective statistical analysis of coagulation parameters after 250 liver transplantations. *Semin Thromb Hemost* 1993;19(3):223-232.

6. Ho KS, Lashner BA, Emond JC, Baker AL. Prior esophageal variceal bleeding does not adversely affect survival after orthotopic liver transplantation. *Hepatology* 1993,18(1):66-72.

7. Langnas AN, Marujo WC, Stratta RJ, et al. Influence of a prior portosystemic shunt on outcome after liver transplantation. *Am J Gastroenterol* 1992;87(6)714-718.

8. Brems JJ, Hiatt JR, Kellin AS, et al. Effect of a prior portosystemic shunt on subsequent liver transplantation. *Ann Surg* 1989;209:51-56.

9. Menegaux F, Keeffe EB, Baker E, et al. Comparison of transjugular and surgical portosystemic shunts on the outcome of liver transplantation. *Arch Surg* 1994;129:1018-1023.

10. Somberg KA. The NIDDK liver transplantation database: transjugular intrahepatic portosystemic shunts (TIPS) have a limited impact on the liver transplant operation. *Gastroenterology* 1994;106(A)989. Abstract.

11. Munoz SJ, Ballas SK, Moritz MJ, et al. Perioperative management of fulminant and subfulminant hepatic failure with therapeutic plasmapheresis. *Transplant Proc* 1989;21:35.

12. Wszolek ZK, McComb RD, Pfeiffer RF, et al. Pontine and extrapontine myelinolysis following liver transplantation. *Transplantation* 1989; 48(6)1006-1012.

13. VonKaulla KN, Kaye H, VonKaulla E, et al. Changes in blood coagulation. *Arch Surg* 1966;92:71.

14. Kang Y. Coagulation in liver transplantation. *Transplant Proc* 1993;25(2):2001-2005.

15. Darby JM, Stein K, Grenvik A, et al. Approach to management of the heart-beating brain-dead organ donor. *JAMA* 1989;261:222.

16. Kang Y, Lewis JH, Navalgund A, et al. Epsilon-aminocaproic acid for treatment of fibrinolysis during liver transplantation. *Anesthesiology* 1987;66:766-773.

17. Pohdorietky, Landers DF, Peters RK, Langnas AN, Shaw BW Jr. The effect of epsilon-aminocaproic acid on blood usage in orthotopic liver transplantation: a double-blind prospective study. Presented at the 19th Annual Meeting of the American Society of Transplant Surgeons, May 1993. Abstract.

Methodologies to Avoid Bleeding in Transplant Surgery

Wolf Bechstein, MD

Gabriele Himmelreich, MD

Hanno Riess, MD

Hemostatic disturbances either may correlate with the magnitude of a surgical procedure – as in heart, lung, pancreas, and kidney transplantation – or may be organ specific, as in bone marrow or liver transplantation. In bone marrow transplantation, there may be tissue damage after conditioning. Prolonged pancytopenia may occur, especially in the setting of concomitant sepsis. Among the solid-organ transplants, uremic thrombocytopathy may present a challenge in kidney transplantation. In heart transplantation, disturbances in hemostasis may be due to preexisting hemostatic defects caused by prior aspirin or other drug therapy or related to the clinical setting of bridging; to transplantation with an artificial heart or ventricular assist device; or to factors intrinsic to the procedure's extracorporeal circulation, eg, hemodilution, autocoagulation, foreign-surface interactions, and hypothermia. Aprotinin use in heart transplantation has been shown to significantly reduce both 24-hour and 48-hour blood loss and, even more important, to significantly reduce the need for nonautologous blood.[1] The most problematic disturbances in hemostasis occur with liver transplantation. Factors involved include difficulties that may be confronted in other surgical procedures in patients with liver cirrhosis: extreme hypersplenism, preexisting increased fibrinolysis, muscle wasting, venous collaterals, portal vein thrombosis, and extensive scarring from previous procedures. Other difficulties are specific to the liver transplant setting: complete cessation of clotting-factor synthesis and loss of clearance function for mediators of fibrinolysis during the anhepatic stage of the procedure, use of venovenous bypass, and possible release of proteinases from the graft, causing hyperfibrinolysis.[2]

In Berlin, we have performed more than 700 liver transplants since our program began in 1988. We used aprotinin in all transplants, except for the first 10. Aprotinin is a serine protease inhibitor with a broad spectrum, inhibiting trypsin, plasmin, kallikrein, and factors XI and XII, among other factors. It causes contact-phase inhibition, with anticoagulant and antifibrinolytic effects at doses of >200 KIU/mL. It has plasmin inhibitor and possibly platelet-protective effects at doses of <150 KIU/mL.

Early studies clearly had shown that hemostasis in liver transplantation is related to the phenomenon of hyperfibrinolysis, occurring especially during the anhepatic phase and immediately after reperfusion.[3] In our first study, we retrospectively compared results in our first 10 patients, transplanted without aprotinin, with results in our next 10 consecutive patients, who were given aprotinin as a bolus of 0.5 million KIU 3 times intraoperatively.[4] Transfusion requirements, including the need for red packed cells and fresh-frozen plasma, were significantly reduced in the aprotinin group, as was the duration of surgery after reperfusion (Table 1). During the postreperfusion phase of surgery, more time is spent on hemostasis than on reconstruction of the bile duct, so the time required for hemostasis clearly was less in patients who had received aprotinin than in those who had not.

Table 1. Effects of Aprotinin on Blood Loss and Duration of Surgery After Reperfusion

	Group 1 (n=10) (w/o Aprotinin)	Group 2 (n=10) (w. Aprotinin)	*P*-value*
RBCs transfused (U)	7.9	3.5	<.05
FFP transfused (U)	9.6	4.4	<.05
FSP (mg/L)	53.6	29.9	
DOS/reperfusion to closure (min)	141	101	<.05
Abdominal DL (mL)	1209	784	
Relaparotomies for hemorrhage (n)	2/10	0/10	

* Mann-Whitney U-test. RBCs. Red blood cells; FFP, fresh-frozen plasma; FSP, fibrinogen split products; DL, drainage loss; DOS, duration of surgery.
(Reprinted with permission from *Lancet*. 1989;ii:924-925, The Lancet Ltd,)

Our experience with the first 46 patients who received aprotinin as a bolus of 3 times 0.5 million KIU intraoperatively was reported in 1991.[5] The average transfusion requirement in these patients was 7.5 red blood cell (RBC) units; this compared with 9.7 units in the 10 patients previously transplanted without aprotinin. Other reported studies, all but one retrospective studies and many using historic controls, mostly showed a similar benefit with aprotinin (Table 2).[6-8] The only prospective controlled study, including only 20 patients, showed no difference in RBC substitution between the aprotinin and control groups.[9]

Table 2. Blood-Product Requirements and Aprotinin in Liver Transplantation

Reference	Treatment	Control	Total Aprotinin Dose (mio KIU)
Bechstein 1991	7.5	9.7	1.5
Grosse 1991	8.1	23.3	5.0
Mallet 1991	7.5	23.6	5.6
Groh 1992	18.0	20.0	5.0
Himmelreich 1992	7.0	8.0	2.0

(Reprinted with permission from *Semin Thrombosis and Hemostasis,* 1993;19:262, Thieme Medical Publishers, Inc.)

Aprotinin use clearly involves a dose factor. The Himmelreich study that was done in our group shows that results differ with different aprotinin regimens.[8] This study compared the effects of aprotinin given by bolus and by infusion. Patients in the bolus group received 0.5 million KIU of aprotinin on induction of anesthesia, at the start of the anhepatic phase, and then at reperfusion. Patients in the infusion group were started with an infusion of 0.2 million KIU immediately after induction of anesthesia which was increased to 0.4 million KIU at the beginning of the anhepatic phase and kept at this level until skin closure. Infusion continued at 0.1 million KIU for 72 hours after the procedure. Heparin was given postoperatively in this study to prevent the advent of feared thromboembolic complications. We no longer administer heparin during the first 24 hours, and the decision to use heparin subsequently is based on the patient's clinical status, with no experience of thromboembolic complications.

Blood sampling was done immediately preoperatively during the induction of anesthesia, 5 minutes before the start of the anhepatic phase, 10 minutes after the start of the anhepatic phase, and then at fixed intervals after reperfusion. The perfusate, consisting of the blood mixed with a preservation solution that emerges as the first flush out of the graft, also was analyzed.

Administration of aprotinin by infusion achieved higher blood levels of aprotinin than administration by bolus, particularly with the higher infusion dose given during the anhepatic phase and reperfusion (Fig 1). Plasminogen levels were significantly lower in the infusion group during the pre-anhepatic phase. There was no significant difference between the two groups in levels of plasmin-antiplasmin complexes (Fig 2). Within the first 8 hours after reperfusion, there were no significant differences between plasminogen activator inhibitor (PAI) levels of both groups.

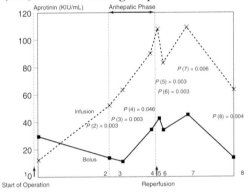

Fig 1. Comparison of bolus and infusion methods of administration on mean aprotinin levels achieved in the blood of patients undergoing liver transplant.

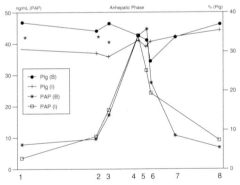

Fig 2. Median concentrations of plasmin-antiplasmin (PAP) complex and plasminogen (Fig) during liver transplantation when aprotinin was given as bolus (B) or by infusion (I). * = $P < 0.05$; B vs I. (Reprinted with permission from *Seminars in Thrombosis and Hemostasis.* 1993;19:197-208, Thieme Medical Publishers Inc)

Perhaps surprisingly, aprotinin also had effects on parameters of leukocyte activation, indicating the presence of aprotinin anti-inflammatory properties.[10] Figure 3 shows levels of elastase-proteinase inhibitor (EPI) complex in both groups; EPI levels were significantly elevated in the infusion patients compared with the bolus patients.

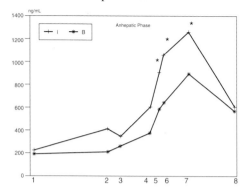

Fig 3. Median concentration of elastase in complex with α-proteinase inhibitor (EPI) during liver transplantation in patients with aprotinin application as bolus (B) or by infusion (I). * = P < 0.01; B vx l. (Reprinted with permission from *Seminars in Thrombosis and Hemostasis.* 1993;19:197-208, Thieme Medical Publishers Inc.)

Analysis of the perfusate for a variety of coagulation and fibrinolysis factors showed significant differences between the two groups in levels of PAI complex and α_2-antiplasmin (Table 3), suggesting that aprotinin also may have a protective effect on the endothelial lining of the graft immediately after reperfusion.

Table 3. Comparative Analysis of the Perfusate of Two Groups of Aprotinin-Treated Liver Transplant Patients

	Median (B) Median (I)	Range (B) Range (I)	P (B/I)
t-PA activity (IU)	12 5	0.7 - 23.6 .7 - 17.4	.101
t-PA antigen (ng/mL)	12.3 10.1	7.2 - 26.6 1.2 - 19.3	.050
PAI activity (AU)	6.4 17.8	0.0 - 22.0 8.8 - 30.4	.043
α_2-antiplasmin (%)	63 93	5.0 - 95.0 68.0 - 102.0	.010
Plasminogen (5)	43 50	3.0 - 77.0 35.0 - 87.0	.288
Fibrinogen (g/L)	1.5 1.5	0.0 - 2.2 0.0 - 2.6	.476
TAT (mg/mL)	93.2 73.5	40.5 - 324.0 32.5 - 1500.0	.288
PC (%)	9.5 15	0.0 - 24.0 3.0 - 50.0	.063
AT-III (%)	31 37	3.0 - 56.0 9.0 - 55.0	.476
C1-inhibitor (%)	65 73	6.0 - 92.0 34.0 - 109.0	.254

B, Bolus, I, infusion; t-PA, tissue plasminogen activity; PAI, plasminogen activator inhibitor; AT-III, antithrombin III. (Reprinted with permission from Williams and Wilkins. Comparison of different hemostatic parameters in the perfusate of 13 patients, *Transplantation* 1992;53:132-136.)

The differences observed with different regimens of aprotinin show that it definitely has effects on parameters of fibrinolysis. The clinical relevance of these effects was studied in a smaller group of patients by comparing blood-product requirements in 13 patients who received the IV bolus regimen and 10 patients who received the continuous IV infusion regimen.[8] There was no significant difference between the two groups in their need for packed red cells (Table 4). This may be attributed both to the small number of patients in this study and to the small amount of packed red cells (8 units) required, even by those patients who received the bolus regimen. Given aprotinin for 72 hours after surgery, the infusion group required significantly less packed red cells than the bolus patients during that period.

**Table 4. Comparison of Blood-Product Requirements in
Bolus versus Continuous Infusion Aprotinin**

	Bolus	Continuous	P
Patients (n)	13	10	
RBC intraop	8	7	NS
FFP intraop	10.5	8	NS
RBC, POD 3	3.5	1.5	<.05
FFP, POD 3	9.5	6.5	NS

RBC, Red blood cells; FFP, Fresh-frozen plasma; NS, not significant; POD, Postoperative day.
(Reprinted with permission from Williams and Wilkins. Blood Produce Requirements in Randomized Trial Himmelreich G, et al., *Transplantation* 1992;52:132.)

A more telling difference in effect between the two aprotinin regimens was observed by analysis of whole-blood lysis as derived from thromboelastograms, which provide a global parameter of fibrinolysis. In this analysis, a time difference of more than 120 minutes between the maximum amplitude of the thromboelastogram to the complete flat line after fibrinolysis indicates the absence of hyperfibrinolysis, between 90 and 120 minutes indicates mild hyperfibrinolysis, and less than 90 minutes indicates severe hyperfibrinolysis. In the bolus group, more than half of all patients showed either mild or severe hyperfibrinolysis. There was only one patient in the infusion group with hyperfibrinolysis, which was severe (Fig 4). Thus, the higher blood levels of aprotinin achieved with the infusion regimen, while not causing a very obvious reduction in blood-product use compared with the bolus regimen, clearly resulted in less hyperfibrinolysis. It can be concluded that aprotinin does prevent fibrinolysis during orthotopic liver transplantation, reducing the frequency and degree of hyperfibrinolysis.

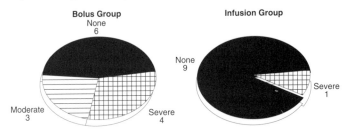

Fig 4. Difference in effect of bolus vs infusion aprotinin regimens in 2 groups of patients as seen by analysis of whole blood lysis from thromboelastogram (WBLT). WBLT > 120 minutes: no hyper-fibrinolysis; WBLT < 120 minutes and > 90 minutes: moderate hyperfibrinolysis; WBLT < 90 minutes: severe hyperfibrinolysis.

Possible side effects of aprotinin include anaphylactic reactions, especially after previous exposure. However, in our series of more than 700 liver transplants, including more than 50 retransplants among patients previously exposed to aprotinin, no anaphylactic reactions occurred. Although thrombotic complications are possible, none attributable to aprotinin occurred in our series. However, there has been a reported case of pulmonary embolism attributed to aprotinin in a liver transplant patient who had received a high dose.[11]

References

1. Havel M, Owen An, Simon P, et al. Decreasing use of donated blood and reduction of bleeding after orthotopic heart transplantation by use of aprotinin. *J Heart Lung Transplant* 1992;111:348-349.

2. Bechstein WO, Riess H, Blumhardt G, et al. Aprotinin in orthotopic liver transplantation. *Semin Thromb Hemost* 1993;19:262-267.

3. Porte RJ, Bontempo FA, Knot EAR, Lewis JH, Kang YG, Starzl TE. Systemic effects of tissue plasminogen activator-associated fibrinolysis and its relation to thrombin generation in orthotopic liver transplantation. *Transplantation* 1989;47:978-984.

4. Neuhaus P, Bechstein WO, Lefebre B, Blumhardt G, Slama K. Effect of aprotinin on intraoperative bleeding and fibrinolysis in liver transplantation. *Lancet* 1989;ii:924-925.

5. Bechstein WO, Riess H, Neuhaus P, et al. The effect of aprotinin on blood-product requirements during orthotopic liver transplantation. *Clin Transplant* 1991;5:422-426.

6. Grosse H, Lobbes W, Frambach M, von Broen O, Ringe B, Barthels M. The use of high-dose aprotinin in liver transplantation: the influence on fibrinolysis and blood loss. *Thromb Res* 1991;63:287-297.

7. Mallet SV, Cox D, Burroughs AK, Rolles K. The intraoperative use of Trasylol (aprotinin) in liver transplantation. *Transplant Int* 1991;4:227-230.

8. Himmelreich G, Muser M, Neuhaus P, Bechstein WO, et al. Different aprotinin applications influencing hemostatic changes in orthotopic liver transplantation. *Transplantation* 1992;53:132-136.

9. Groh J, Welte M, Azad SC, Forst H, Pratzschke E, Kratser MAA. Does aprotinin affect blood loss in liver transplantation? *Lancet* 1992;340:173.

10. Riess H, Jochum M, Machleidt W, Himmelreich G, Bechstein WO, et al. Role of leukocytes in hemostasis during orthotopic liver transplantation. *Semin Thromb Hemost* 1993;19:197-208.

11. Baubillier E, Cherqui D, Dominique C, et al. A fatal thrombotic complication during liver transplantation after aprotinin administration. *Transplantation* 1994;57:1664-1666.

Workshop III:
New Aspects of
Hemostatic Transfusion

Mechanisms Regulating Surgical Hemostasis

Laurence A. Harker, MD

Normally, nonreactive endothelium interfaces with highly reactive elements circulating in blood from highly-thrombogenic constitutents in the subendothelium. The hemostatic apparatus comprises complex interactive processes involving endothelium, platelets, coagulation, and fibrinolysis (Fig 1).[1-3] Immediately after surgical injury, platelets and plasma coagulation factors interact with subendothelial connective tissue structures, initiating the production of thrombin and the formation of localized hemostatic plugs.

Surgical disruption of tissues exposes adventitial cell-bound tissue factor (TF) to plasma coagulation factor VII/VIIa, producing a tight TF:FVIIa complex that catalytically activates factors IX and factor X locally on phospholipid platelet surfaces, leading to the explosive production of thrombin via enzyme-cofactor complexes (Figs 1 and 2). Thrombin activates platelets and cleaves fibrinogen and factor XIII, giving rise to fibrin-stabilized hemostatic plugs.

Platelets attach to nonendothelialized surfaces under high-shear conditions via von Willebrand factor that is bound to subendothelial matrix, present in plasma, and secreted by adjacent intact endothelium and deposited platelets.[4] The process of attaching activates platelets, thereby inducing the expression of functional receptors for fibrinogen and other adhesive proteins from membrane glycoprotein IIb/IIIa (GPIIb/IIIa) integrin by altering its conformation.[5,6] Platelet cohesion depends on establishing fibrinogen linkages between adjacent activated platelets.

Ambient platelets are recruited by activation through three independent, yet interrelated, agonists: (1) Thrombin, generated on phospholipid surfaces, activates the platelet thrombin receptor by cleaving its extracellular aminoterminus;[7] (2) adenosine diphosphate (ADP), secreted from platelet storage granules, initiates receptor signaling; and (3) thromboxane A_2 (TxA_2), arising via platelet arachidonic acid metabolism, induces platelet receptor activation (Fig 1).

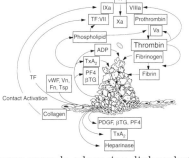

Fig 1. Platelets adhere to subendothelial connective tissue elements at sites of endothelial disruption, primarily through von Willebrand factor (vWF) ligand formation between platelet receptor glycoprotein Ib (GPIb) and subendothelial collagen. Adhesive proteins, fibronectin (Fn), vitronectin (Vn), and thrombospondin (Tsp) may also participate in adhesion to subendothelium through platelet receptors GPIIb/IIIa and GPIV. Platelet adhesion initiates a series of complex interactive platelet recruitment reactions comprising (1) release of dense-granule adenosine diphosphate (ADP); (2) activation of platelet membrane phospholipase complex to form thromboxane A2 (TxA2); and (3) release of α-granule-binding proteins, including fibrinogen, vWF, Fn, Vn, and Tsp. Platelet recruitment requires expression of GPIIb/IIIa as a ligand receptor. Generally, platelet-platelet binding occurs through calcium-dependent bridging with fibrinogen. βTG, β-thromboglobulin; PDGF, platelet-derived growth factor; PF4, platelet factor 4. (Modified from *Baillière's Clinical Haematology*: 1994;7:500.)

Thrombin is the principal mediator of platelet recruitment in the formation of hemostatic plugs. The structure of thrombin reveals its catalytic active site and binding domains. All of the functions of thrombin are dependent on its catalytic activity; substrate specificity is determined by the flanking binding domains. Thrombin binds with fibrin in the hemostatic plug.[8] Bound thrombin retains its catalytic ability to activate platelets and cleave fibrinogen, but is resistant to the inhibitory effects of heparin because the heparin-binding domain on thrombin is not available after binding with fibrin in the hemostatic plug.[9]

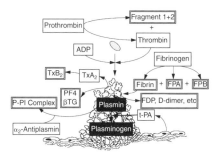

Fig 2. Intravascular extension of thrombus is limited by multiple protective mechanisms, the most important of which are related to the presence of thrombin and/or intact endothelium and include (1) inactivation by complex formation with plasma antithrombin III (AT-III); (2) facilitation by endothelial heparin-like molecules of the inactive thrombin:antithrombin III complex formation; and (3) downregulation of thrombin formation through destruction of surface-bound factor VIIIa and factor Va by activated protein C (Act PC) formed by thrombomodulin-dependent thrombin cleavage, and thrombin-mediated release from endothelium of tissue plasminogen activator (t-PA), prostacyclin (PGI2), and nitric oxide (NO-). Additionally, intact endothelium adjacent to forming thrombus inactivates adenosine diphosphate (ADP) and vasoactive amines released from activated platelets. (Modified from *Baillière's Clinical Haematology*:1994;7:500.)

Thrombin converts fibrinogen to soluble fibrin monomer by removing fibrinopeptide A. The hemostatic plug becomes stabilized by the formation of insoluble fibrin strands through fibrin polymerization and cross-linking via the transpeptidase activity of thrombin-activated factor XIII.[1]

Tissue factor is the pivotal factor initiating thrombin generation at sites of vascular disruption.[10] The exposure/expression of tissue factor bound to tissues, and not free in circulating blood, guarantees localized hemostatic responses, thereby safeguarding intact adjacent blood vessels from the threat of developing thrombo-occlusive complications. Additional processes limiting the extension of hemostatic plug formation include: (1) rapid binding of thrombin to thrombomodulin on intact endothelium, leading to the production of activated protein C and its subsequent inactivation of activated factor V, a critical cofactor in thrombin production; (2) thrombin-induced endothelial generation of antiaggregatory prostacylin and nitric oxide, together with enhanced secretion of tissue plasminogen activator (t-PA) and (3) inactivation of excess thrombin by endothelial heparin-like glycosaminoglycans, leading to enhanced neutralization of excess soluble thrombin by plasma antithrombin.[1]

Hemostatic plugs, consisting of adherent and coherent platelets, insoluble cross-linked fibrin, leukocytes, and entrapped red cells, undergo gradual removal by progressive local conversion of plasminogen to plasmin by activation of plasminogen activators within the hemostatic plug, followed by plasmin-mediated catalysis of fibrin.[11] This thrombolytic process is regulated by the relative rates of plasminogen activation and inactivation via natural inhibitors, including plasminogen activator inhibitor-1 (PAI-1) and plasma antiplasmin. The full thrombolytic activity expressed by t-PA depends on binding with fibrin to optimize its confirmation for fibrin cleavage. Moreover, bound t-PA resists inhibition by PAI-1.[12] Additionally, plasmin bound to fibrin is protected from inactivation by circulating α_2-antiplasmin.[13] The continuing utilization of platelets and fibrinogen during the postoperative period reflects the active fibrinolytic removal and reformation of hemostatic plugs during the early healing process.[1,14]

Bound plasmin is inhibitable by the serine protease inhibitor aprotinin and the lysine analogues ε-aminocaproic acid (EACA) and tranexamic acid (AMCHA), thereby protecting the hemostatic plug from endogenous thrombolysis.[15] Accordingly, the administration of plasmin antagonists throughout surgical procedures reduces surgical blood loss, even if hemostatic plug formation may be impaired, eg, in the instance of thrombocytopenia or hemophilia.

DEFECTIVE SURGICAL HEMOSTASIS

Since the consequences of failed surgical hemostasis are so great, it is important to identify genetic and acquired disorders preoperatively by thoughtful inquiry into the outcome of prior hemostatic challenges, family history, associated diseases, and concurrent medications. Additionally, appropriate laboratory screening of platelet, coagulation, and fibrinolytic functions are required for surgical procedures imposing significant challenge to the hemostatic apparatus. The recommended screening tests involve assessing platelet hemostatic function (platelet count and template bleeding time); coagulation (thrombin time, prothrombin time, and partial thromboplastin time); and fibrinolysis (D-dimer levels and whole-blood or euglobulin lysis time). The template bleeding time is a useful clinical test for assessing overall platelet hemostatic plug-forming capability (Fig 3).[16]

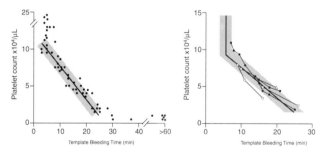

Fig 3. Inverse relation of bleeding time to circulating platelet count in patients with thrombocytopenia on the basis of impaired production when the concentration of platelets is between 10,000 and 100,000 per microliter. Regression line is shown by the solid line, and 95% confidence limits are indicated by the shaded area. (Modified from *Baillière's Clinical Haematology*: 1994;7:500.)

Cardiovascular surgery impairs hemostasis by: (1) reducing the circulating concentration of hemostatic blood constituents by diluting with buffer used to prime the bypass and oxygenator apparatus (Fig 4); (2) progressively inhibiting platelet hemostatic function secondary to the effects of the artificial surfaces comprising the bypass and oxygenator apparatus, hypothermia, and various drugs administered during bypass surgery (Fig 5); and (3) enhancing removal of hemostatic plugs by activating fibrinolysis.[15,17] Thus, defective hemostasis may lead to abnormal surgical bleeding because of short-lived hemostatic plugs due to early lysis and rebleeding, as well as because of inherent inability to form primary hemostatic plugs. Accordingly, bleeding during cardiac surgery may be excessive, and occasionally disastrous.

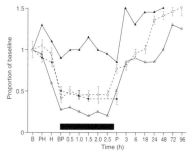

Fig 4. Nonblood prime in the extracorporeal oxygenator bypass dilutes the red cells and albumin to about half (solid circles). Circulating fibrinogen levels (open circles) are similarly decreased by dilution, as are the prothrombin complex factors (II, VII, IX, and X). Coagulation factor V (open triangles) is reduced in excess of dilution and factor VIII (closed triangles) levels are relatively unaffected by dilution. Clotting factor levels return to baseline values or above within 12 h after bypass. Horizontal solid bar indicates period of bypass. Error bars represent ± 1 SE.

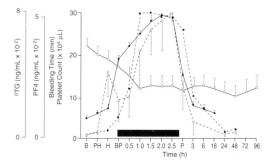

Fig 5. Platelet count (open triangles) falls progressively during initial operative and bypass period, in part due to dilution by nonblood priming solutions. Thereafter the platelet count remains about half baseline, exceeding 100,000 platelets/µl l throughout the 4-day period of observation. Bleeding time (solid circles) is unaffected by heparinization but increases abruptly after the initiation of bypass and lengthens progressively during the first 2 h of bypass, at which time it is >30 min. Plasma PF4 (open circles) peaks sharply after heparinization, followed by a progressive rise throughout remainder of bypass. Plasma β-thromboglobulin (closed triangles) levels rise rapidly after initiation of bypass to maximum levels at 1 h. Bleeding time measurements, PF4, and β-TG fall quickly after bypass. Horizontal solid bar identifies the period of bypass. Error bars represent + 1 SE.

Aspirin Use and Blood Loss: The VA Experience

Aspirin increases surgical blood loss when given to patients undergoing cardiovascular surgery. The most convincing data regarding the effect of aspirin on blood loss associated with saphenous vein aortocoronary bypass surgery come from the prospective placebo-controlled randomized clinical trials involving more than 900 men included in the Veterans Administration Cooperative Studies Program.[18-21] In these studies, aspirin (325 mg daily) prior to cardiopulmonary bypass (CPB) surgery increased 35-hour median chest-tube drainage from 805 mL to 965 mL (P= 0.02) (Fig 6). A three-fold increase in the dose of aspirin (325 mg tid) further increased chest-tube drainage to 1175 mL (P= 0.01); three-time daily aspirin in combination with dipyridamole resulted in 1000 mL of chest-tube drainage (P= 0.02). Chest-tube blood loss in all aspirin groups was 1035 mL (P< 0.001 compared with placebo). The blood loss was evenly distributed among all the patients in the aspirin groups and was not due to a few patients who bled heavily.

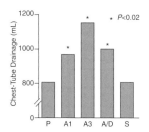

Fig 6. Blood loss data obtained from 35-h postoperative chest-tube drainage. Values are medians. P, Placebo; A1, aspirin once daily; A3, aspirin three times daily; A/D, aspirin/dipyridamole; S, sulfinpyrazone. *P<.02 refers to comparison between each treatment group and placebo. (Reproduced with permission from *Circulation* 1988;77:1329.)

There was no change in the overall pattern of blood loss over the course of the study. Patients given preoperative aspirin also received more transfusions of red blood cells and platelet concentrates than the placebo control group (P< 0.005). Additionally, the reoperation rate in the aspirin groups exceeded that in the groups not receiving aspirin (P< 0.01). In the follow-up study, the VA investigators also demonstrated that initiating aspirin therapy within hours postoperatively (as opposed to preoperatively) produced equivalent antithrombotic benefits (P= 0.871) and less operative bleeding.[22,23]

Aspirin Use and Blood Loss: Other Studies

Other published experience supports the conclusion that aspirin increases blood loss in patients undergoing cardiovascular surgery. In a retrospective study the estimated odds-ratio for reoperation due to abnormal bleeding was 1.82 in patients receiving aspirin compared with patients not ingesting aspirin within 7 days prior to cardiovascular surgery.[24] In another study, the duration of chest-tube drainage for nonaspirin patients was 20 hours, compared with 34 hours for patients receiving aspirin (P<0.001). Conversely, patients not receiving aspirin until 1 to 4 days postoperatively showed no evidence of increased bleeding when compared with nonaspirin control patients.[25,26] By contrast, perioperative aspirin failed to measurably increase operative or postoperative surgical bleeding in association with other surgical procedures, including hip and knee surgery.[27-29] Convincing evidence from clinical trials establishes the corollary conclusion that the usual hemorrhagic complications arising during acute and chronic aspirin therapy are attributable to the dose-dependent local erosive effects of aspirin on the gastro-intestinal mucosa.[30]

These findings indicate that the blockade of TxA_2 by systemic aspirin induces insufficient impairment in platelet hemostatic function to produce significant surgical bleeding, unless additional hemostatic aberrations are also present, such as transient platelet dysfunction due to CPB, heparin or warfarin-type anticoagulation, or thrombolytic therapy. Thus, the TxA_2 pathway of platelet recruitment is of minimal importance compared with the aspirin-independent thrombin pathway in hemostatic plug formation after tissue injury.[8,31] Excessive bleeding after surgery occurs when the formation of platelet plugs is defective, either due to thrombocytopenia or to platelet dysfunction; for example, effects of drugs (such as aspirin or ticlopidine), effects of cardiovascular devices (such as oxygenator apparatus),[32] or effects of hereditary platelet defects. When defective hemostasis is secondary to quantitative or qualitative platelet disorders, excessive surgical bleeding is successfully treated by transfusional platelet replacement. Thus, aspirin therapy does not increase the risks of excessive surgical bleeding except in patients undergoing CPB or with associated defects/therapies that disrupt the hemostatic mechanism. Since the increase in surgical bleeding produced by aspirin in patients undergoing cardiovascular surgery is relatively small and readily treatable, it is seldom necessary to delay such surgery when the indications are compelling and urgent.

Ticlopidine-Associated Bleeding Risks
Understanding the risks of surgical bleeding in patients receiving ticlopidine therapy is much more problematic than in the case of aspirin because of ticlopidine's antiplatelet properties and the sparsity of reliable clinical data. Although it is not precisely known how ticlopidine inhibits platelet function, it is established that ticlopidine blocks the final common pathway in platelet recruitment, ie, dose-response inhibition of the functional fibrinogen receptor expression mediating platelet cohesion. Thus, ticlopidine globally impairs platelet responses to all agonists/pathways of activation (Fig 1). Because ticlopidine must be taken orally for several days to exhibit antiplatelet activity and because none of its metabolites have direct antiplatelet activity and its inhibitory effects persist throughout the lifespan of platelets, it is postulated that ticlopidine irreversibly impairs platelet membrane-signaling mechanisms during megakaryocyte/platelet development.[17,33] Therefore, ticlopidine, as opposed to aspirin, has a dose-dependent antihemostatic effect, as evidenced by ticlopidine's dose-dependent prolongation of the template bleeding time.

Accordingly, excessive surgical bleeding should be expected in patients receiving ticlopidine therapy in proportion to the degree of platelet dysfunction produced by the dose administered, ie, prolongation of the template bleeding time.

While this direct association between intensity of antiplatelet effect and bleeding complications is clinically borne out with other GPIIb/IIIa-dependent global antagonists of platelet recruitment, information regarding the effects of perioperative ticlopidine therapy after cardiovascular surgery is sparse.[22,34-37] However, there are controlled clinical trials assessing chronic ticlopidine therapy demonstrating that it significantly increases the risk of spontaneous bleeding,[38-40] including purpura, epistaxis, hematemesis, and melena. Thus, on the basis of available information, it appears that achieving both efficacy and safety for ticlopidine, as opposed to aspirin, involves dose titration to produce intermediate antiplatelet effects, ie, 10- to 15-minute bleeding time demonstrating the presence of antiplatelet activity without abolishing platelet hemostatic competence. For the majority of patients, the currently recommended dose of 250 mg twice daily accomplishes that goal. However, this approach indicates that any surgical procedures performed in patients receiving therapeutic doses of ticlopidine will implicitly be associated with at least some increase in the risk of excessive bleeding, even in the absence of additional hemostatic abnormalities. Thus, ticlopidine is predicted to have a greater predisposition to excessive surgical bleeding than aspirin, although the available scant clinical reports do not yet confirm this postulate.

Impaired Coagulation-Associated Surgical Bleeding
Abnormal bleeding also develops when activation of the coagulation cascade is impaired by either factor deficiency or factor inhibition, eg, hemophilia or heparin therapy. The clinical screening tests for detecting defective coagulation includes the thrombin time, prothrombin time (PT), and activated partial thromboplastin time (aPTT).

Fibrinolysis-Associated Surgical Bleeding
Excessive fibrinolysis also leads to surgical bleeding, as illustrated by hemorrhagic events complicating therapeutic thrombolysis or by spontaneous bleeding associated with hereditary reduction in natural antifibrinolytic inhibitors, eg, deficiencies in α_2-antiplasmin or PAI-1. Global screening tests for assessing fibrinolysis include various modifications of the euglobulin lysis time or the whole-blood clot lysis test.

PREVENTING ABNORMAL SURGICAL BLEEDING BY INHIBITING FIBRINOLYSIS
Because hemostasis may be impaired by either defective formation or inadequate retention of hemostatic plugs, it follows that excessive surgical bleeding secondary to defects in hemostasis may be prevented by transfusional replacement of the reduced or defective factor, or by delaying fibrinolytic removal of already formed hemostatic plugs by inhibiting plasmin or its formation.

Clinical trials in several different settings support the approach of preventing abnormal surgical bleeding by inhibiting fibrinolysis in the presence of defective hemostasis. First, abnormal bleeding is prevented in hemophiliacs undergoing dental surgery by administering EACA or AMCHA orally before and after the surgical procedure. Second, chronic oral EACA or AMCHA also reduces spontaneous gastrointestinal bleeding in patients with thrombocytopenia secondary to marrow failure. Third, the inhibition of plasmin during cardiac surgery by administering intravenous aprotinin substantially reduces surgical bleeding.

Thus, excessive surgical bleeding secondary to impaired hemostatic plug formation may be largely prevented by delaying the fibrinolytic removal of already formed hemostatic plugs.

LOCAL CORRECTION OF ABNORMAL SURGICAL BLEEDING
Defective hemostasis may lead to abnormal surgical bleeding because of short-lived hemostatic plugs due to early lysis and rebleeding, as well as be-

cause of inherent inability to form primary hemostatic plugs. Accordingly, surgical bleeding during cardiac surgery is usually excessive, and sometimes disastrous.

Abnormal hemostatic plugs may be prone to early lysis because of defective fibrin substrate; excessive release of plasminogen activator(s) from adjacent stimulated vascular tissues and healing tissues; and excessive infiltration and release of proteolytic enzymes from leukocytes. Surgical intervention, trauma, or extracorporeal circulation may have opposing effects on the rate at which hemostatic plugs undergo lysis: (a) enhanced local fibrinolysis due to increased release of plasminogen activators from endothelium; or (b) enhanced vascular release of protease inhibitors.

REFERENCES

1. Harker LA, Mann KG. Thrombosis and fibrinolysis. In Fuster V, Verstraete M (eds): *Thrombosis in Cardiovascular Disorders.* Philadelphia, WB Saunders Co; 1992;1-16.

2. Colman RW, Hirsh J, Marder V, Salzman EW. *Hemostasis and Thrombosis: Basic Principles and Clinical Practice.* Philadelphia, Pa: JB Lippincott; 1994.

3. Harker LA. Pathogenesis of thrombosis. In: Williams WJ, Beutler E, Erslev AJ, Lichtman MA, eds. *Hematology.* New York, NY: McGraw-Hill; 1990:1559-1569.

4. Fressinaud E, Baruch D, Rothschild C, Baumgartner HR, Meyer D. Platelet von Willebrand factor: evidence of its involvement in platelet adhesion to collagen. *Blood* 1987;70:1214-1217.

5. Kieffer N, Phillips DR. Platelet membrane glycoproteins: functions in cellular interactions. *Annu Rev Cell Biol* 1990;6:329-357.

6. Ruoslahti E. Integrins. *J Clin Invest* 1991;87:1-5.

7. Vu T-KH, Hung DT, Wheaton VI, Coughlin SR. Molecular cloning of a functional thrombin receptor reveals a novel proteolytic mechanism of receptor activation. *Cell* 1991;64:1057-1068.

8. Harker LA, Maraganore JM, Hirsh J. Novel antithrombotic agents. In: Colman RW, Hirsh J, Marder VJ, Salzman EW, eds: *Hemostasis and Thrombosis: Basic Principles and Clinical Practice.* Philadelphia, Pa: JB Lippincott;1994: 1638-1660.

9. Weitz JI, Hudoba M, Massel D, Maraganore J, Hirsh J. Clot-bound thrombin is protected from inhibition by heparin-antithrombin III but is susceptible to inactivation by antithrombin III-independent inhibitors. *J Clin Invest* 1990;86:385-391.

10. Harker LA, Kelly AB, Hanson SR. Antithrombotic benefits and hemorrhagic risks. *Thromb Haemost* 1995;74:464-472.

11. Collen D, Lijnen HR. Basic and clinical aspects of fibrinolysis and thrombolysis. *Blood* 1991;78:3114-3124.

12. Collen D, Lijnen HR. Molecular and cellular basis of fibrinolysis. In: Hoffman R, Benz EJ, Jr., Shattil SJ, Furie B, Cohen HJ, eds. *Hematology: Basic Principles and Practice.* New York, NY: Churchill Livingstone; 1991:1232-1242.

13. Weitz JI, Leslie B, Hirsh J, Klement P: $\alpha 2$-antiplasmin supplementation inhibits tissue plasminogen activator-induced fibrinogenolysis and bleeding with little effect on thrombolysis. *J Clin Invest* 1993;91:1343-1350.

14. Harker LA, Slichter SJ. Platelet and fibrinogen consumption in man. *N Engl J Med* 1972;287:999-1005.

15. Salmenpera MT, Levy JH, Harker LA. Hemostasis and cardiopulmonary bypass. In: Guyton RA, Finlayson DC, Rigatti RL, eds: *Cardiopulmonary Bypass: Principles and Techniques of Extracorporeal Circulation*. New York, NY: Springer-Verlag; 1995:88-113.

16. Harker LA, Slichter SJ. The bleeding time as a screening test for evaluation of platelet function. *N Engl J Med* 1972;287:155-159.

17. Woodman RC, Harker LA. Bleeding complications associated with cardiopulmonary bypass. *Blood* 1990;76:1680-1697.

18. Goldman S, Copeland J, Moritz T, Henderson W, Zadina K, Ovitt T, et al. Improvement in early saphenous vein graft patency after coronary artery bypass surgery with antiplatelet therapy: results of a Veterans Administration Cooperative study. *Circulation* 1988;77:1324-1332.

19. Henderson W, Moritz T, Goldman S, Copeland J, Souchek J, Zadina K, et al. The statistical analysis of graft patency data in a clinical trial of antiplatelet agents following coronary artery bypass grafting. *Controlled Clin Trials* 1988;9:189-205.

20. Goldman S, Copeland J, Moritz T, Henderson W, Zadina K, Ovitt T, et al. Saphenous vein graft patency 1 year after coronary artery bypass surgery and effects of antiplatelet therapy. *Circulation* 1989;80:1190-1197.

21. Henderson W, Goldman S, Copeland J, Moritz T, Harker L. Antiplatelet or anticoagulant therapy after coronary artery bypass surgery. A meta-analysis of clinical trials. *Ann Intern Med* 1989;111:743-750.

22. Caliendo G, Bradbury K, Mehl B. Ticlopidine, bleeding, and surgery. *Mt Sinai J Med* 1994;61:372-373.

23. Goldman S, Copeland J, Moritz T, Henderson W, Zadina K, Ovitt T, et al. Starting aspirin therapy after operation: effects on early graft patency. *Circulation* 1991;84:520-526.

24. Bashein G, Nessly ML, Rice AL, et al: Preoperative aspirin therapy and reoperation for bleeding after coronary artery bypass surgery. *Arch Intern Med* 1991;151:89-93.

25. Lorenz RL, Weber M, Kotzur J, et al. Improved aortocoronary bypass patency by low-dose aspirin (100 mg daily): effects on platelet aggregation and thromboxane formation. *Lancet* 1984;1:1262-1264.

26. McEnany MT, Salzman EW, Mundth ED, et al. The effect of antithrombotic therapy on patency rates of saphenous vein coronary artery bypass grafts. *J Thorac Cardiovasc Surg* 1982;83:81-89.

27. Harris WH, Salzman EW, Athanasoulis C, et al. Comparison of warfarin, low-molecular-weight dextran, aspirin, and subcutaneous heparin in prevention of venous thromboembolism following total hip replacement. *N Engl J Med* 1977;297:1246-1249.

28. Powers PJ, Gent M, Jay RM, et al. A randomized trial of less intense postoperative warfarin or aspirin therapy in the prevention of thromboembolism after surgery for fractured hip. *Arch Intern Med* 1989;149:771-774.

29. Hull R, Delmore TJ, Hirsh J, et al. Effectiveness of intermittent pulsatile elastic stockings for the prevention of calf and thigh vein thrombosis in patients undergoing elective knee surgery. *Thromb Res* 1979;16:37-45.

30. Hirsh J, Dalen JE, Fuster V, Harker LA, Salzman EW. Aspirin and other platelet-active drugs: the relationship between dose, effectiveness and side effects. *Chest* 1992;102:327S-336S.

31. Hanson SR, Harker LA. Interruption of acute platelet-dependent thrombosis by the synthetic antithrombin D-phenylalanyl-L-prolyl-L-arginyl chloromethylketone. *Proc Natl Acad Sci USA* 1988;85:3184-3188.

32. Harker LA, Malpass TW, Branson HE, Hessel I, Slichter SJ. Mechanism of abnormal bleeding in patients undergoing cardiopulmonary bypass: acquired transient platelet dysfunction associated with selective alpha granule release. *Blood* 1980;56:824-834.

33. Harker LA, Gent M. Antiplatelet agents in the management of thrombotic disorders. In: Colman RW, Hirsh J, Marder VJ, Salzman EW, eds. *Hemostasis and Thrombosis: Basic Principles and Clinical Practice.* Philadelphia, Pa: JB Lippincott; 1994:1506-1513.

34. The EPIC Investigators. Use of a monoclonal antibody directed against the platelet glycoprotein IIb/IIIa receptor in high-risk coronary angioplasty. *N Engl J Med* 1994;330:956-961.

35. Harker LA. Platelets and vascular thrombosis. *N Engl J Med* 1994;330:1006-1007.

36. Limet R, David J-L, Magotteaux P, Larock M-P, Rigo P. Prevention of aorta-coronary bypass graft occlusion: beneficial effect of ticlopidine on early and late patency rates of venous coronary bypass grafts: a double-blind study. *J Thorac Cardiovasc Surg* 1987;94:773.

37. Chevigne M, David J-L, Rigo P, Limet R. Effect of ticlopidine on saphenous vein bypass patency rates: a double-blind study. *Ann Thorac Surg* 1984;37:371.

38. Hass WK, Easton JD, Adams HP. A randomized trial comparing ticlopidine hydrochloride with aspirin for the prevention of stroke in high-risk patients. *N Engl J Med* 1989;321:501.

39. Gent M, Blakely JA, Easton JD. The Canadian American Ticlopidine Study (CATS) in thromboembolic stroke. *Lancet* 1989;1:1215.

40. Janzon L, Bergqvist D, Boberg J, et al. Prevention of myocardial infarction and stroke in patients with intermittent claudication: effects of ticlopidine. Results from STIMS, the Swedish Ticlopidine Multicentre Study. *Scand J Int Med* 1990;227:301.

Methods for Recognizing the Patient at Risk of Perioperative Bleeding

Colin R.M. Prentice, MD, FRCP

Failure to secure full, effective hemostasis is the most common cause of perioperative bleeding. After surgery, generalized vasodilation occurs, and at this stage there may be extensive bleeding and oozing from wound surfaces that can amount to significant blood loss. In such cases, there may be no identifiable coagulation or platelet defect.

There are, however, patients with a true bleeding tendency that may be due to an inherited coagulation disorder, such as hemophilia A or B, or to an acquired disorder that may be related to the condition for which surgery is required. Careful preoperative screening makes it possible to recognize the vast majority of these patients who will be at risk of excessive hemorrhage during surgery.

ROUTINE PREOPERATIVE SCREENING

Table 1 details the routine screening that is part of the preoperative assessment at our institution to identify at-risk patients.

Table 1. Routine Preoperative Screening

History

Clinical examination

Urea, electrolytes

Liver function tests

Repeat history after lab tests

Platelet count

Activated partial thromboplastin time

Prothrombin time

Patient History

History of previous bleeding in the patient should be sought. In particular, a bleeding tendency may be indicated by spontaneous bleeding such as epistaxis or hematuria, gastrointestinal bleeding, or inappropriately severe bleeding or bruising after minor trauma or previous surgery. Details of any transfusions necessary for bleeding should be obtained. Questions should then concentrate on any family history of bleeding, especially in male relatives such as uncles, cousins, or grandparents, remembering that inherited diseases such as hemophilia can skip a generation if there are female carriers in the preceding generation.

Drug Usage

A large number of drugs can affect bleeding and the normal hemostatic response to surgery. Patients on oral anticoagulants need to be identified. Aspirin and nonsteroidal anti-inflammatory agents are commonly prescribed drugs that will affect platelet function by inhibiting thromboxane A_2 (TxA_2).[1] Although some clinicians stop aspirin therapy prior to surgery, some patient populations (for example, those undergoing coronary artery bypass graft surgery) may still be taking aspirin at the time of surgery. Another group of patients frequently taking aspirin preoperatively are those undergoing orthopedic procedures who are at risk of deep-vein thrombosis postoperatively. We have studied over 3500 patients at our institution and in collaboration with centers in Australia and New Zealand and have not seen any deleterious effects of aspirin treatment in these patients undergoing complex orthopedic procedures.[2]

Clinical Examination and Laboratory Tests

Routine laboratory tests of urea, electrolytes, and liver function will identify underlying illnesses such as renal and hepatic diseases that may predispose a patient to bleeding. Occasionally, severe systemic disorders such as sepsis or malignancy may give rise to disseminated intravascular coagulation (DIC).

Platelet Function

Platelet count is an extremely important routine investigation to conduct, as platelet deficiency (thrombocytopenia) will increase bleeding tendency. Patients with such deficiency may give a history of easy bruising, bleeding from the gums, epistaxis, melena, or hematuria. On examination, they may show areas of excessive bruising or petechiae. Normal platelet function is a central event in the response to endothelial injury. The primary event in the hemostatic plug formation is the binding of the platelet glycoprotein 1b receptor (GP1b) to von Willebrand factor (vWF), which originates from the exposed subendothelium. This complex of vWF and GP1b plays a critical role in platelet adhesion, and an abnormality in this receptor complex may result in bleeding tendencies. For the platelet plug to develop, platelet activation and aggregation must occur. Collagen and thrombin are potent platelet activators, whereas adenosine diphosphate (ADP), epinephrine, prostaglandin endoperoxides, platelet activating factor (PAF), serotonin, and TxA_2 are weaker agonists.

Thrombocytopenia may result from bone marrow suppression as a consequence of leukemia or cytotoxic drug therapy; or the patient may suffer from idiopathic thrombocytopenia purpura, a condition in which the platelet count can fall below 20,000.[3] Platelet destruction can also occur as part of the overall picture of DIC.[4] In this condition, infective or antigenic insults to the vascular endothelium give rise to increased expression and release of tissue factor, leading to circulating tissue factor/factor VIIa complex, which initiates coagulation. This causes, within the blood stream, the formation of microfibrils of fibrin, which are then rapidly broken down to form soluble fibrin/fibrinogen fragments known as fibrin degradation products (FDP). The depletion of clotting factors and fibrinogen due to intravascular consumption together with the formation of FDP, which have an anticoagulant action, cause a major coagulation disturbance and, in extreme cases, incoagulable blood. It is not surprising that patients so affected have catastrophic hemorrhage, especially in the presence of thrombocytopenia.

Thrombocytopathies are ill-defined, often difficult to recognize disorders in platelet function and can be congenital or acquired. They tend to be rare; examples include Glanzmann's thrombasthenia, 'storage pool defect', and Bernard-Soulier syndrome. von Willebrand's disease, although not a disease of platelet dysfunction, will prolong bleeding time due to defective platelet adhesion to the damaged subendothelial surface, as a result of absent or defective vWF.[5]

Platelet dysfunction can be investigated according to the algorithm shown in Fig 1. A careful patient history and the associated laboratory tests will define how far into the investigative pathway to proceed. This is assessed on an individual patient basis. Many laboratories, our own included, do not proceed to bleeding time estimation if the platelet count is normal. However, a prolonged bleeding time will warrant further investigation and will often be associated with a deficiency in vWF and factor VIII. This picture of von Willebrand's syndrome is nearly always congenital but can be acquired. A normal vWF leads to platelet aggregability studies that can diagnose the rare hereditary disorders of platelet function.

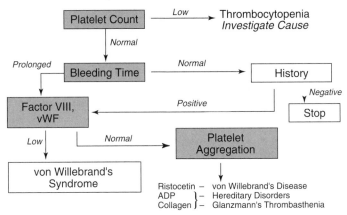

Fig 1. Flow chart of laboratory tests that can be used to assess impaired hemostasis due to platelet dysfunction. Investigations should be conducted on an individual patient basis and in conjunction with a careful history. vWF, von Willebrand factor; ADP, adenosine diphosphate.

Coagulation Function Measurement

Activated partial thromboplastin time (aPTT) and prothrombin time (PT) are measures of the intrinsic (contact phase) and extrinsic pathways of the coagulation cascade, respectively, both of which result in the generation of factor Xa. The reaction then proceeds along a common pathway, resulting in the generation of thrombin, which converts fibrinogen to insoluble fibrin clot (Fig 2).

Fig 2. Intrinsic (contact phase) and extrinsic pathways of the coagulation cascade both result in generating factor Xa. The contact activation phase of coagulation begins with the generation of active Hageman's factor (factor XIIa), which in turn converts factor XI to factor XIa. Factor IX activated by factor XIa forms a complex with factor VIII, factor X, phospholipid, and calcium ions to generate factor Xa. The extrinsic route of coagulation starts with the liberation of tissue factor from the endothelium and the formation of a complex with factor VII and calcium ions. The reaction then proceeds along a common pathway that results in generating thrombin, the enzyme that converts fibrinogen to insoluble fibrin clot. TF, Tissue factor; FSP, fibrinogen split products.

Activated Partial Thromboplastin Time

The aPTT mimics intrinsic pathway activation.[6] Citrated blood from the patient is mixed with phospholipid and a surface activator (celite or kaolin), and the reaction is started by the addition of calcium. The contact activation phase of coagulation begins with the generation of active Hageman's factor (factor XIIa), which in turn converts factor XI into factor XIa. The role of factor XIa is to convert inactive factor IX to its active form, and this enzyme together with the cofactor (factor VIII) is responsible for the generation of factor Xa.

A prolonged aPTT will be reported with deficiency in factor VIII and factor IX resulting from the inherited conditions hemophilia and von Willebrand disease.[5] Acquired deficiencies can occur with liver disease (reducing the vitamin K dependent factors IX and X) or if the patient is on oral anticoagulant therapy.[7]

Curiously, one of the commonest causes of prolonged aPTT in our laboratory is the presence of the lupus anticoagulant. The lupus anticoagulant is so called because it was first described in patients with systemic lupus erythematosus (SLE). However, we now know that these autoantibodies are directed against phospholipids and are found over half the time in patients who do not have SLE. Paradoxically, although the lupus anticoagulant is inhibitory in laboratory coagulation tests, it predisposes to *thrombosis* in patients and can be a cause of recurrent abortion. For this reason, patients with a family history of thrombosis, or thrombosis at an early age, should be screened in the laboratory for the lupus anticoagulant.

One -Stage Prothrombin Time

The PT reveals disorders in the extrinsic pathway and is a simple test based on incubation of patient plasma, calcium, and tissue thromboplastin (tissue factor). The addition of tissue factor accelerates the normal clotting time for plasma from 5 minutes to about 10 seconds. In vivo, the extrinsic pathway for factor Xa generation requires the release of tissue factor from the injured endothelial surface. Tissue factor complexes with factor VII in the plasma to form an enzymatic complex that cleaves factor X to factor Xa (Fig 2).

A prolonged PT will again be reported in liver disease if hepatocellular failure reduces the synthesis of factor VII. Malabsorption syndrome, cholestatic jaundice, celiac disease, major gastrointestinal surgery, and blind loop syndrome can all result in vitamin K deficiency and be associated with coagulation dysfunction.[8] In addition, oral anticoagulants will prolong the PT.

Thrombin Clotting Time

Fibrinogen level can be very easily estimated by a thrombin clotting time that evaluates the final stage in the coagulation cascade; namely, the action of thrombin on fibrinogen and clot formation. The time is prolonged in fibrinogen deficiency. There are also numerous methods to estimate fibrinogen levels that are quick and simple to perform.

Fibrin Degradation Products

Plasmin enzymatically degrades fibrin into a number of cleavage fragments (FDP). Marked elevation of FDP levels will be associated with DIC. Plasmin is produced by the action of plasminogen activators: tissue plasminogen activator (t-PA) and urokinase-like plasminogen activator (uPA). During DIC, fibrin is formed inappropriately within the circulation and may persist, causing widespread microvessel thrombosis and multisystem failure, or be cleaved by plasmin into FDP. Thus, FDP serve as a marker for the fibrinolytic dissolution of fibrin and indicate indirectly that fibrin has been formed intravascularly. Normally, a low elevated level of FDP occurs during and after all types of major surgery or trauma. However, marked elevation of FDP indicates that DIC has taken place. If these high levels are associated with a falling fibrinogen level, the presence of uncompensated DIC is inferred.

SUMMARY

Awareness of a bleeding risk in all patients having surgery should cause the surgeon, physician, and anesthetist to screen patients appropriately from the hemostatic aspect. This will undoubtedly reduce the risk of major hemorrhage.

References

1.   Patrono C, Ciabattoni G, Patrignani P, et al. Clinical pharmacology of cyclooxygenase inhibition. *Circulation* 1985;72:1177-1184.

2.   MacMahon S, Rodgers A, Collins R, Farrell B. Antiplatelet therapy to prevent thrombosis after hip fracture. *Br J Bone Joint Surg* 1994;76-B:521-524.

3.   Jackson D. Management of thrombocytopenia. In: Colman R, Hirsh J, Marder V, Salzman E, eds. *Hemostasis and Thrombosis*. 2nd ed. Philadelphia, Pa: Lippincott; 1987:530-536.

4.   Davies J, Grant P. Acquired bleeding disorders. In: Forbes C, Cuschieri A, eds. *Management of Bleeding Disorders in Surgical Practice*. Oxford, England: Blackwell; 1993:46-67.

5.   Sharp R, Forbes C. Inherited bleeding disorders. In: Forbes C, Cuschieri A, eds. *Management of Bleeding Disorders in Surgical Practice*. Oxford, England: Blackwell; 1993:19-45.

6.   Min Hong Saw, Mackie M. Laboratory diagnosis of excess bleeding. In: Forbes C, Cuschieri A, eds. *Management of Bleeding Disorders in Surgical Practice*. Oxford, England: Blackwell; 1993:68-87.

7.   Joist J. Hemostatic abnormalities in liver disease. In: Colman R, Hirsh J, Marder V, Salzman E, eds. *Hemostasis and Thrombosis*. 2nd ed. Philadelphia, Pa: Lippincott; 1987:861-871.

8.   Mannucci P, Giangrande P. Acquired disorders of coagulation. In: Bloom A, Forbes C, Thomas D, Tuddenham E, eds. *Haemostasis and Thrombosis*. 3rd ed. London, England: Churchill Livingstone; 1994:949-968.

Mechanism of Action of Antifibrinolytic Drugs

Colin Longstaff, PhD

Two classes of antifibrinolytic agents have been widely demonstrated to reduce bleeding after surgery or in hemostatic disorders: the small protein serine protease inhibitor aprotinin (also known as bovine pancreatic trypsin inhibitor) and the ω-aminoacids 6-aminohexanoic acid (AHA) or ε-aminocaproic acid (EACA) and tranexamic acid (AMCHA). These agents have different mechanisms of action, although the precise details are still a matter for debate.

APROTININ

Proteases are classified into four enzyme classes: metallo, cysteine, aspartate, and serine. Each of these classes has an associated group of inhibitors. The serine protease enzymes require serine at the active site. They are involved in the coagulation and fibrinolytic cascades and include plasmin, tissue plasminogen activator (t-PA), urokinase (UK), and thrombin.

Aprotinin is a serine protease inhibitor belonging to the Kunitz family, a large group of related inhibitors (tissue factor pathway inhibitor and eglin C, for example). The common mechanism of action of these inhibitors is to form a tight, though reversible, 1:1 stoichiometric complex with the active site of the target enzyme. Aprotinin has been shown to react with many serine proteases (eg, trypsin, plasmin, chymotrypsin, kallikrein, elastase, UK, and thrombin). The range of affinity is very wide, with the inhibition constant (K_i) for trypsin (6 x 10^{-14} M) 500 million-fold less than that for UK or thrombin (around 30 µM). The important reactions with respect to hemostasis are likely to be with plasmin and kallikrein, although plasmin, with a subnanomolar K_i, is likely to be the most important target.

A pivotal event in the control of bleeding is the activation of the coagulation cascade, which culminates in the action of thrombin on fibrinogen to generate fibrin (Fig 1). Fibrin can be maintained by prevention of its fibrinolytic degradation. Plasmin plays a central role in digesting fibrin directly and can operate in a positive feedback loop to generate active two-chain UK from single-chain inactive UK, which then converts plasminogen into plasmin. Plasmin once generated is always in association with fibrin and in normal circumstances is not found free in the circulation due to the action of the naturally occurring serine protease inhibitors α_2-antiplasmin and α_2-macroglobulin.

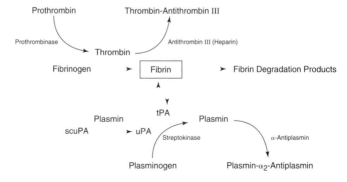

Fig 1. Enzymology of coagulation and fibrinolysis.

A great deal is known about the biochemical and biophysical properties of aprotinin, including the three-dimensional structure.[1] Intermolecular hydrogen bonding and hydrophobic disulfide bridges make this small protein molecule very stable; a large degree of activity will be retained even after boiling. Far less is known about plasmin. The complete amino acid sequence is known, but the overall tertiary structure is not, although structures are published for some kringle domains (see below). Plasmin is made up of two chains, A and B. The B chain contains the active-site pocket, and this is where substrates and aprotinin bind. The A chain contains the regulatory region composed of five kringles that control the interaction of plasmin with other ligands; for example, fibrin and α_2-antiplasmin. Interactions with the A chain may alter the active site in the B chain and affect the way plasmin reacts with substrates and inhibitors.

Plasmin-Aprotinin Kinetics in Solution

Assessment of inhibitor efficacy must take into account not only the level of inhibition achieved but also the rate at which this inhibition takes place. Very tight complexes between enzyme and inhibitor can occur, but if the rate of reaction is slow, in vivo efficacy will be diminished. Fig 2 shows the data for the inhibition of plasmin by aprotinin in solution. Reactions were initiated by adding enzyme (plasmin) to a mixture of plasmin-specific chromogenic substrate (*p*-nitroanilide) and inhibitor (aprotinin) and monitoring the production of chromophore production in a spectrophotometer. Over time, the rate of substrate hydrolysis declines as more enzyme is complexed by inhibitor. Plots of optical density versus time can then be fitted by nonlinear regression analysis. Two equations were used to fit the data: equation 1 (dashed line in Fig) for generation of chromophore with irreversible enzyme-inhibitor binding or equation 2 (solid line in Fig) where enzyme-inhibitor binding is reversible. It can be seen from Fig 2 that the best fit for the data was with equation 2, indicating that the inhibitory action of aprotinin on plasmin was reversible. By conducting a series of experiments over a range of inhibitor concentrations at constant substrate and enzyme concentrations (*inset,* Fig 2), it is possible to derive the inhibition constant for the reaction. Inhibition constants (K_i) can be calculated from the slope of a plot of Vmax/*vs* versus [I], where Vmax is the plasmin activity at saturating chromogenic substrate and *vs* is the steady-state rate of substrate hydrolysis at equilibrium with inhibitor; [I] is the inhibitor concentration (*see section below*).[2]

Fig 2. Slow-binding inhibition curves for binding of aprotinin to plasmin. Main curve shows the hydrolysis of 0.5 nM plasmin of 0.9 mM chromogenic substrate in the presence of 20 nM aprotinin. Reactions were monitored for 5 hours. Inset shows a family of curves obtained in similar experiments over a range of concentrations of inhibitor. (5, 10, 20, 40, 60 nM) to produce curves showing more inhibition. (Reprinted with permission from *Blood Coagulation and Fibrinolysis,* Vol 3, 1994.)

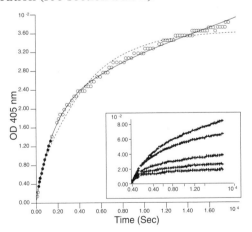

Plasmin-Inhibition Constants in the Presence of Kringle Binding Ligands

Plasmin inhibition by aprotinin has been studied in the presence of a number of plasmin effectors known to interact with kringle-binding sites and modulate plasmin activity against substrates and inhibitors.[3] Plasmin was incubated with a chromogenic substrate and the presence or absence of the kringle-binding ligands AMCHA, AHA, and CNBr-fibrinogen fragments. Inhibition by aprotinin over the concentration range 0.5 nM to 100 nM was studied in microtiter plates and optical density monitored to follow the progress of inhibition by aprotinin. Inhibition constants were calculated from the slopes of plots of Vmax/vs versus [I], where Vmax is the plasmin activity at saturating chromogenic substrate and vs is the steady state rate of substrate hydrolysis at equilibrium with inhibitor; [I] is the inhibitor concentration (Fig 3).[4] The slope of the line is $1/K_i$. The steeper the slope, the lower the K_i (better inhibition). It can be seen that the presence of the kringle binding ligands had an insignificant influence on the binding of aprotinin and plasmin. The mean inhibition constant from these results was 0.44 nM. In contrast, these ligands would have had significant effects on plasmin binding to the naturally occurring inhibitors α_2-antiplasmin or α_2-macroglobulin.

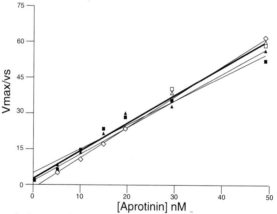

Fig 3. Inhibition of plasmin by aprotinin in free solution in the presence of kringle-binding ligands. Plasmin was allowed to reach equilibrium in the presence of increasing concentrations of aprotinin with no effector (O), 100 µM tranexamic acid (•), 500 µM tranexamic acid (□), 1 mM tranexamic acid (■), 25 nM aminohexanoic acid (△), 8 µg/mL CNBr-fibrinogen fragments (▲), 20 µg/mL fibrinogen fragments (◊). (Reprinted with permission from *Blood Coagulation and Fibrinolysis*, Vol 5, 1994.)

Reaction of Aprotinin With Fibrin-Bound Plasmin

It is important to remember that most studies to determine inhibition constants are carried out with purified systems in free solution as described above. An important question to address is whether aprotinin remains an effective plasmin inhibitor in vivo when the plasmin activity is associated with fibrin.

A fibrin clot lysis method has been developed to monitor plasmin activity in the presence of fibrin.[3] Fibrinogen was clotted with thrombin in microtiter plates to produce an opaque clot in each well. Plasmin was added to fibrin clots containing increasing concentrations of aprotinin and the rate of clot lysis monitored as decreasing optical density. Figure 4 shows the results of plasmin-catalysed fibrin clot lysis from two separate experiments in the presence of aprotinin. Rates of lysis in the presence of inhibitor are expressed as percentage of rate with no inhibitor and demonstrate 50% inhibition of lysis occurring around 2 nM aprotinin.

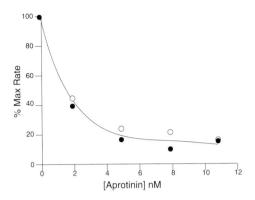

Fig 4. Inhibition of plasmin digestion of fibrin clots by aprotinin. Results indicate that 50% inhibition of lysis occurs around 2 nM. Open and closed symbols represent data from two separate experiments. (Reprinted with permission from *Blood Coagulation and Fibrinolysis*, Vol 5, 1994.)

Inhibition was less effective than in pure solution ($K_i \approx 0.4$ nM), which can be accounted for by fibrin acting as a substrate in competition for the active site of the enzyme. Therefore, there appear to be no significant effects of kringle-fibrin interactions, in agreement with the studies performed in pure solutions (*see* above). These data indicate that aprotinin is still a very potent inhibitor of plasmin even in the presence of fibrin. It should also be stressed that other enzyme-substrate interactions will raise apparent K_i values, ie, make aprotinin a poorer inhibitor in vivo compared with studies in pure systems. Thus, the possible interactions of aprotinin with kallikrein and other proteases are weaker in vivo than expected from the quoted figures determined in pure systems in vitro.

Reaction of Aprotinin With Cell Receptor-Bound Plasmin

Both plasminogen and plasmin can bind to cell-surfaces, and plasminogen receptors have been investigated on many cell types.[5,6] Studies using human umbilical vein endothelial cells and rat C6 glioma cells in culture have demonstrated that cell-associated plasmin is protected from inhibition by α_2-antiplasmin as well as α_2-macroglobulin.[7] Therefore, it is possible that plasmin bound to ubiquitous receptors, protected from physiologic inhibitors, could also be protected from aprotinin. This was investigated using Nalm6 cells (a pre-B leukemic cell line).

Nalm6 cells are known to express cell-surface plasminogen receptors and are useful, as they have very low intrinsic fibrinolytic activity, with no release of UK or t-PA.[8] Experiments similar to those previously described using fibrin were performed with cells to investigate the inhibitory action of aprotinin on plasmin bound to these cell-surface receptors. Over a wide range of cell concentration (high receptor density), aprotinin was able to inhibit the bound plasmin effectively (unpublished data). Therefore, it seems plasmin bound to either fibrin or cell receptors is protected from physiologic inhibitors but remains susceptible to aprotinin.

SYNTHETIC ANTIFIBRINOLYTIC AGENTS

The synthetic antifibrinolytic agents AHA (or EACA) and AMCHA are closely related to the amino acid lysine. The primary mode of action of these ω-aminoacids as antifibrinolytic agents is usually ascribed to their ability to block the lysine-binding sites (kringles) of plasmin(ogen) and t-PA, which are the domains responsible for binding these molecules to fibrin and cells.[9] Tranexamic acid is approximately 10 times more potent than AHA in vitro due to the cyclohexane ring that fixes a stable structure with maximal effectiveness. At very high concentrations, these ω-aminoacids are able to block the active site of plasmin, but these concentrations are not achieved in vivo with the doses of agents used. However, another mechanism of action proposed for AHA is that this analogue can bind to fibrin and in some way protect it from plasmin digestion.[10,11] This remains to be demonstrated conclusively.

Reaction of Tranexamic Acid and Aprotinin With Fibrin-Bound Plasmin

Data presented above show the lysine analogues act via kringles and do not affect aprotinin binding to plasmin (Fig 3). The combination of aprotinin and AMCHA could, therefore, have additive or even synergistic effects on plasmin activity. Experiments were performed to study the effects of these two agents in combination.[3] The fibrin clot lysis method described previously was used. Aprotinin up to 5 nM was incorporated into fibrin clots and the effect of additional AMCHA (50 μM, 100 μM, 150 μM) on plasmin-catalysed clot lysis was recorded (Fig 5). Figure 5 *inset* shows a plot of the aprotinin concentration required at each AMCHA concentration to achieve 75% inhibition of clot lysis rate. A linear diagonal plot (dotted line) indicates that the two agents were additive, whereas curves below the diagonal suggest synergistic behavior.[12] These data imply an additive effect with possibly a small degree of synergy.

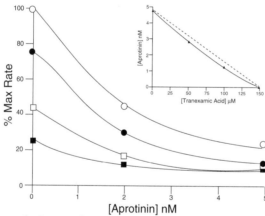

Fig 5. Inhibition of plasmin lysis of fibrin clots in the presence of aprotinin and tranexamic acid. Tranexamic acid concentrations were none (O), 50 μM (•), 100 μM (□), 150 μM (■). Inset shows the aprotinin concentration required at each tranexamic acid concentration to achieve 75% inhibition of the rate of fibrin lysis. Dotted line is the expected plot for a purely additive relationship; concave curve below this line indicates synergy. (Reprinted with permission from *Blood Coagulation and Fibrinolysis*, Vol 5, 1994.)

SUMMARY

Although aprotinin and ω-aminoacids both act by different mechanisms, it is likely that interactions with plasmin play a key role in their physiologic activities. Plasmin is a key enzyme in fibrinolysis, and the affinity of plasmin for aprotinin is high. Plasmin inhibition directly reduces digestion of fibrin, and can reduce feedback activation of plasminogen and plasminogen activators (UK and t-PA) and prevent digestion and depletion of α_2-antiplasmin. The significance of plasmin inhibition by aprotinin in preserving platelets is still unclear. Although it is also argued that kallikrein inhibition may explain some of the clinical effects of aprotinin administration, this has not been demonstrated convincingly, since aprotinin is a poorer inhibitor of kallikrein and kallikrein has a smaller role in fibrinolysis than plasmin.

References

1. Gebhard W, Tschesche H, Fritz H. Biochemistry of aprotinin and aprotinin like inhibitors. In: Barratt A, Salvesen G, eds. *Proteinase Inhibitors*. Oxford,UK: Elsevier; 1986:375-388.

2. Longstaff C, Gaffney PJ. Studies on the mechanism of binding of serpins and serine proteases. *Blood Coagul Fibrinolysis* 1992;3:89-97.

3. Longstaff C. Studies on the mechanisms of action of aprotinin and tranexamic acid as plasmin inhibitors and antifibrinolytic agents. *Blood Coagul Fibrinolysis* 1994;5:537-542.

4. Longstaff C, Gaffney P. Serpin serine protease binding kinetics: α_2-antiplasmin as a model inhibitor. *Biochemistry* 1991;30:980-986.

5. Plow E, Felez J, Miles L. Cellular regulation of fibrinolysis. *Thromb Haemost* 1991;66:32-36.

6. Hajjar K. Cellular receptors in the regulation of plasmin generation. *Thromb Haemost* 1995;74:294-301.

7. Hall SW, Humphries JE, Gonias SL. Inhibition of cell surface receptor-bound plasmin by $alpha_2$-antiplasmin and alpha2-macroglobulin. *J Biol Chem* 1991;266:12329-12336.

8. Felez J, Chanquia C, Fabregas P, Plow E, Miles L. Competition between plasminogen and tissue plasminogen activator for cellular binding sites. *Blood* 1993;82:2433-2441.

9. Iwamoto M. Plasminogen-plasmin system IX: specific binding of tranexamic acid to plasmin. *Thromb Diath Haemost* 1975;33:573-585.

10. Urano S, Metzger A, Castellino F. Plasmin-mediated fibrinolysis by variant recombinant tissue plasminogen activators. *Proc Natl Acad Sci USA* 1989;86:2568-2571.

11. Maxwell R, Allen D. Interactions of ε-aminocaproic acid with the thrombin clotting and fibrinolytic systems. *Nature* 1966;209:211-213.

12. Reed G, Matsueda G, Haber E. Synergistic fibrinolysis: combined effects of plasminogen activators and an antibody that inhibits α_2-antiplasmin. *Proc Natl Acad Sci USA* 1990;87:1114-1118.

Anti-Inflammatory Effects of Serine Protease Inhibitors

Jawed Fareed, PhD, Michael Koza, BS,
Jeanine M. Walenga, PhD, Debra Hoppensteadt, PhD,
Roque Pifarré, MD

Endogenous serine protease inhibitors (SERPINs) play an important role in regulating proteases to maintain balance in the coagulation, fibrinolysis, complement cascade, and kallikrein-kinin systems.[1-3] These inhibitors regulate thrombogenesis, excessive fibrinolysis, generation of hypotensive mediators such as bradykinin, anaphylotoxins, and protease digestible products. Some of the major SERPINs and their physicochemical characteristics are shown in Table 1, which also depicts the relative plasmatic levels of each. Antithrombin III (AT-III) is one of the major inhibitors of thrombin and other procoagulant enzymes, whereas α_2-antiplasmin controls fibrinolysis. C1 esterase inhibitor is capable of controlling the activation of kallikrein and C1 esteroprotease. This inhibitor, therefore, has an important role in the control of hemodynamic aberrations due to the activation of kallikrein and the complement-mediated pathways.

Physicochemical Characteristics of Major SERPINs			
Inhibitors	**MW**	**Concentration** **μM**	**Enzymes Inhibited**
α_1-Antitrypsin	55,000	35-71	Trypsin, chymotrypsin, plamin, thrombin, collagenase, elastase
Antithrombin III	65,000	3.5-6.3	Thrombin, kallikrein, factor IXa, factor Xa, factor XIa, factor XIIa
Heparin cofactor II	60,000	1.0-3.0	Thrombin
α_2-macroglobulin	725,000	2.0-5.8	Trypsin, chymotrypsin, plasma kallikrein, thrombin, elastase
PAI	Various	Various	Plasminogen activator
α_2-Antiplasmin	65,000	1.5-1.8	Plasmin
α_2-Antichymotrypsin	69,000	4.4-8.7	Chymotrypsin
Inter a-trypsin	160,000	1.2-4.4	Trypsin, chymotrypsin (weak) inhibitor
C1 Inactivator	104,000	1.4-3.3	Factor XIa, factor XIIa, kallikrein
TFPI*	34,000	<0.01	

* Increased 10 to 20-fold after heparinization. SERPINs, Serine protease inhibitors; MW, molecular weight; PAI, plasminogen activator inhibitor; TFPI, tissue factor pathway inhibitor.

More recently, tissue factor pathway inhibitor (TFPI) has been recharacterized as an important inhibitor of the extrinsic pathway.[4-6] While in the resting state, the levels of this inhibitor are relatively low (<0.01 nm); after heparinization, the circulating levels are increased up to two-fold.[7] The exact role of this increase in the TFPI level in the control of thrombogenesis and other protease pathways is not known.

The structures of the tissue factor and TFPI are compared in Fig 1. Tissue factor is a transmembrane protein and is primarily responsible for thrombin generation. This activator also has several other properties, including activation of cells and modulation of the vascular system. In contrast to tissue factor, TFPI is a polydomain inhibitor with multiple inhibitory properties. This protein modulates both the plasmatic and cellular responses, as well as modulating factor VII-mediated activation of the clotting process. Furthermore, it can also inhibit the activation of platelets during endovascular injury. Thus, during the heparinization process when large amounts of this inhibitor are released, tissue factor-mediated pathways can be controlled by the release of TFPI. Besides inhibiting the clotting process, TFPI is also known to inhibit the procoagulant process and leukocytic enzymes. Thus, this inhibitor plays multiple roles in the control of the pathophysiology of thrombotic disorders. It may also play a modulatory role in the inflammatory process. The Kunitz-3 domain resembles aprotinin in structure. As shown in Fig 2, there is a structural resemblance between aprotinin and TFPI. Thus, when used in conjunction with heparin, aprotinin's effects may be augmented due to the release of TFPI.

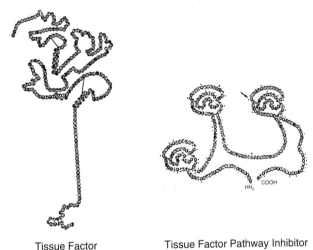

Tissue Factor   Tissue Factor Pathway Inhibitor

Fig 1. Comparison of the primary structure of tissue factor with tissue factor pathway inhibitor (TFPI). Tissue factor is a transmembrane protein with both plasmatic and tissue-factor receptor activation properties. TFPI selectively inhibits tissue factor and its mediated responses. Thus, in addition to controlling coagulation activation, this inhibitor is also involved in the control of inflammatory responses.

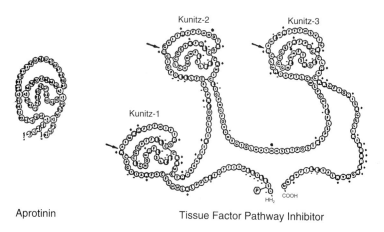

Kunitz-2

Kunitz-3

Kunitz-1

HH₂ COOH

Aprotinin

Tissue Factor Pathway Inhibitor

Fig 2. Comparison of the structures of aprotinin and TFPI. Both are classified as Kunitz-type inhibitors. Aprotinin is a broad-spectrum protease inhibitor, whereas TFPI inhibits factor Xa, tissue factor-factor VIIa complex, and elastase. The tissue factor-factor VIIa complex and elastase inhibitory actions of aprotinin and TFPI may be mutually synergistic.

Tissue factor pathway inhibitor is capable of producing strong inhibition of factor VIIa and factor Xa. Chymotrypsin and plasmin are also inhibited to a lesser extent. However, at concentrations of up to 100 µg/mL, it does not produce inhibition of amidolytic actions of kallikrein, activated protein C, tissue plasminogen activator (t-PA), urokinase, thrombin, and streptokinase-plasminogen complex (Fig 3). The complete biochemical and pharmacologic profile of TFPI is unknown. With the availability of recombinant TFPI, it is now possible to investigate the actions of this inhibitor.

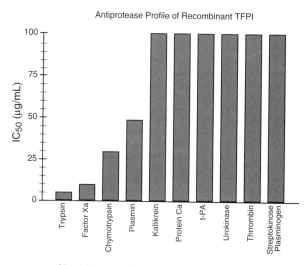

Antiprotease Profile of Recombinant TFPI

Fig 3. Antiprotease profile of recombinant TFPI as measured by using synthetic substrate-based methods. These studies were carried out in purified enzyme systems.

Some of the potential targets for the anti-inflammatory effects of SERPINs include inhibition of the activation of factor XIIa, kallikrein, and plasmin; inhibition of the release and activity of polymorphonuclear neutrophils (PMN) elastase; and interactions with other endogenous protease inhibitors such as TFPI. These effects of SERPINs may result in modulating cellular and plasmatic sites that can facilitate anti-inflammatory responses.

A comparison of the structure of recombinant aprotinin and recombinant hirudin shows that both exhibit similar molecular-weight profiles (Fig 4). While aprotinin inhibits plasmin and kallikrein, its effects on thrombin are almost insignificant. Recombinant hirudin, however, produces a strong and specific inhibition of thrombin. Both agents are in clinical development for various indications.

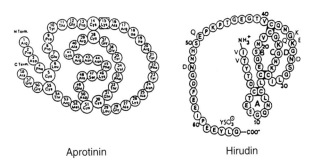

Aprotinin   Hirudin

Fig 4. Comparison of the primary structures of aprotinin and hirudin. Both proteins have similar molecular weights; both are now produced by recombinant technology. Aprotinin is a broad-spectrum inhibitor, whereas hirudin is monospecific.

Table 2 shows a list of various enzymes that are inhibited by aprotinin and the relative physiologic consequences of its inhibition. As can be seen, aprotinin produces relatively potent inhibition of kallikrein, plasmin, and factor XIIa. All of these enzymes in some ways are involved in the mediation of inflammatory responses. Thus, modulation of serine proteases plays a role in controlling inflammation. On the other hand, inhibition of other enzymes also helps in hemostatic restoration and control of fibrinolysis.

Table 2. Enzymes Inhibited by Aprotinin

Enzyme	Degree of Inhibition	Physiologic Consequences
Plasma kallikrein	4+	Inhibition of coagulation and kinin generation
Glandular kallikrein	4+	Inhibition of kinin generation
Factor XIIa	3+	Inhibition of coagulation, fibrinolysis, clotting process
Tissue factor/factor VIIa	1+	Inhibition of clotting process
Plasmin	3+	Inhibition of thrombolysis
Plasminogen activator	1-3+	Inhibition of thrombolysis
Protein Ca	1+	Hemostatic restoration; inhibition of thrombolysis
C1-Esterase	2+	Anti-inflammatory action
Neutrophil elastase	1+	Anti-inflammatory action
Cathepsins	+	Cellular modulation

By direct or indirect mechanisms, aprotinin also modulates certain cellular sites, involving PMN leukocytes, macrophages, endothelial cells, fibroblasts, smooth-muscle cells, and platelets. Such modulatory actions also help in the cytorestoration and control of bleeding and other pathologic processes (Table 3).

Table 3. Modulation of Cellular Responses by Aprotinin

Cells	Modulation
Polymorphonuclear	Inhibition of granulocytic enzymes; cytostabilization
Macrophages	Inhibition of tissue factor and granulocytic enzymes
Endothelial cells	Inhibition of t-PA; cytostabilization
Fibroblasts	Unknown
Smooth-muscle cells	Modulation of contractile actions (NO mediated?)
Platelets	Cytoprotection; inhibition of endopeptidase; probable NO-mediated regulation

t-PA, Tissue plasminogen activator; NO, Nitric oxide.

Aprotinin itself is capable of producing synergistic and additive interactions with other serine proteases (Table 4). Aprotinin may produce different degrees of interactions with serine proteases. For example, its interactions with α_2-antiplasmin may be helpful in controlling bleeding, and its interaction with TFPI may be useful in controlling thrombogenesis and white cell-mediated inflammatory responses.

Table 4. Aprotinin Interactions With SERPINs

SERPIN	Interaction
Antithrombin III	Unknown
Heparin cofactor II	Unknown
Plasminogen activator inhibitor	Additive
α_2-Antiplasmin	Synergistic
α_2-Macroglobulin	Additive
α_1-Antitrypsin	Additive
C1 Esterase inhibitor	Additive
Tissue factor pathway inhibitor	Synergistic

SERPINs, serine protease inhibitors.

Aprotinin is often administered during cardiovascular surgical procedures. In this indication, heparinization results in a measurable release of TFPI (Table 5).[8] Heparinization results in up to a four-fold increase in TFPI levels, which may modulate the actions of tissue factor released from surgical sites. Thus, tissue factor-mediated activation of both plasmatic and cellular sites can be altered.

Table 5. Tissue Factor Pathway Inhibitor Release During Cardiovascular Bypass Surgery

Group	TFPI (ng/mL)
Baseline	110 ± 20
Post-heparinization	630 ± 68
Post-protamine neutralization	190 ± 26

All results represent the mean $\pm$ 1 SD of 10 individual cases. TFPI antigen was measured. TFPI, Tissue factor pathway inhibitor; SD, standard deviation.

Aprotinin by virtue of its antiprotease effects may modulate several effects of heparin, including inhibiting VIIa-tissue factor complex, inhibiting factor XIIa activation, altering heparin binding to platelet membranes, and inhibiting heparin-mediated t-PA release. Also, it may produce synergistic effects on the action of TFPI (Table 6). All of these effects may result in decreased bleeding, decreased fibrinolysis, and reduced inflammatory responses.

Table 6. Aprotinin Modulation of Heparin-Mediated Plasmatic and Cellular Effects

Effect	Clinical Outcome
Inhibition of VIIa tissue factor	Decreased activation of tissue factor-complex mediated mechanisms
Inhibition of factor XIIa activation	Control of factor XIIa-mediated protease processes
Reduction of heparin binding to platelet membranes	Platelet function modulation
Inhibition of heparin-mediated t-PA release	Control of thrombolysis-mediated bleeding
Potential synergism of heparin-TFPI-mediated tissue factorTF-VIIa complex inhibition	Control of TF-VIIa-mediated cellular released and plasmatic activation processes

t-PA, Tissue plasminogen activator; TFPI, tissue factor pathway inhibitor; TF, tissue factor.

Polymorphonuclear leukocyte-released elastase may produce sizeable inflammatory effects. The regular Hammersmith dosage of aprotinin results in decreased elastase levels during cardiopulmonary bypass (CPB) surgery. As shown in Fig 5, at various times during cardiovascular surgery, aprotinin produced a decrease in PMN elastase levels. This suggests that aprotinin produces significant effects on PMN to control the PMN release of elastase.

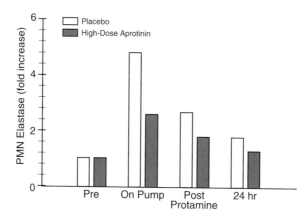

Fig 5. Effect of aprotinin on leukolytic polymorphonuclear neutrophils (PMN) elastase levels during cardiopulmonary bypass surgery as measured by using an immunologic method. All results represent a mean of 3 individual cases.

Bradykinin is one of the important mediators of inflammatory responses, producing multiple effects at various levels. Bradykinin generation during various pathologic states indicates an ongoing inflammatory process. In a study of the effect of high-dose aprotinin on the relative generation of bradykinin, two groups of patients were included. The placebo group (n=10) received no aprotinin, whereas the high-dose aprotinin-treated groups received the Hammersmith regimen. It is noted that a large amount of bradykinin is strongly inhibited by aprotinin. These data are highly suggestive of the anti-inflammatory actions of aprotinin. After protamine neutralization, the differences between the placebo and aprotinin-treated groups are rather minimal (Fig 6).

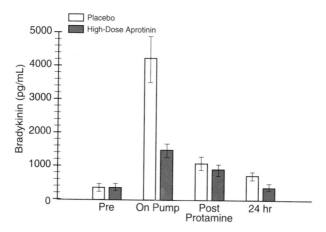

Fig 6. Effect of aprotinin on bradykinin generation during cardiovascular bypass surgery. All results shown here represent a mean ± 1 SD of ten individual cases.

Besides bradykinin, several neuropeptides play a crucial role in mediating pain and inflammatory responses during CPB. Table 7 compares various neuropeptides and bradykinin levels in the control of aprotinin-treated groups at baseline and on pump samples. While procedure-related alterations were observed, the most striking differences in the control and aprotinin-treated groups were found to be in the vasoactive intestinal peptide (VIP) and bradykinin levels. A slight decrease in substance P was also noted. These results indicate that aprotinin primarily modulates the generation of bradykinin, and only minimal effects on the neuropeptides are observed. Additional studies are needed to determine the relative roles of kinins and neuropeptides during cardiovascular surgery. Furthermore, the role of aprotinin in modulating these peptides warrants additional studies.

Table 7. Measurement of Neuropeptides During CPB				
	Control		Aprotinin	
	Pre	On Pump	Pre	On Pump
Neuropeptide Y	6.5 ± 3.2	42.1 ± 8.1	7.8 ± 3.1	36.8 ± 8.1
CGRP	21.4 ± 4.4	26.1 ± 5.3	17.8 ± 4.9	30 ± 8
Substance P	3.5 ± 0.6	48 ± 31	5.6 ± 2.1	36 ± 6.0
Neuropeptide A	5.2 ± 1.3	5.6 ± 0.6	5.8 ± 1.8	6.1 ± 2.1
Neuropeptide B	1.9 ± 0.3	2.9 ± 0.4	2.1 ± 0.8	3.6 ± 2.1
VIP	4.1 ± 0.8	18.4 ± 3.7	5.6 ± 0.9	5.1 ± 2.6
Bradykinin	230 ± 48	2104 ± 54	254 ± 60	1120 ± 210

CPB, Cardiopulmonary bypass; VIP, vasoactive intestinal peptide.

Several synthetic and recombinant inhibitors of serine proteases are currently used for various clinical indications; many of the newer ones are being developed for different cardiovascular and thrombotic indications (Table 8). Aprotinin is an established inhibitor of fibrinolysis and the kallikrein-kinin system and has been used for some time for various medical and surgical indications. Its use as an inhibitor of the fibrinolytic system has added a new dimension to controlling medical and surgical bleeding. Through this application, several additional pharmacologic properties of this agent have been discussed.

Table 8. Synthetic and Recombinant Serine Proteases for Clinical Use

Inhibitor	Clinical Indications	Developmental Status
Aprotinin	Control of fibrinolysis Management of bleeding	Additional indications in medical and surgical areas
EACA	Control of fibrinolysis	Established use in control of bleeding
AMCHA	Control of fibrinolysis	Established use in control of bleeding
Recombinant PAI	Control of fibrinolysis	Experimental use in control of bleeding
C1 Esterase inhibitors	Sepsis, pancreatitis	Limited indications
AT-III	Thrombophilia, DIC, heparin resistance	Anti-inflammatory indications
Heparin cofactor II	Thrombophilia	No additional development
TFPI	Sepsis, thrombophilia	Cardiovascular indications Tissue factor indications
Hirudin	Thrombosis	Adjunct use
Hirulog	Thrombosis	Alternative to heparin
Argatroban	Thrombosis	Heparin-induced thrombocytopenia
Efegatran	Thrombosis	Alternative to heparin
DX 9065a	Thrombosis	Alternative to heparin

EACA, τ-Aminocaproic acid; AMCHA, tranexamic acid; PAI, plasminogen activator inhibitor; AT-III, antithrombin III; DIC, disseminated intravascular coagulation; TFPI, tissue factor pathway inhibitor

More recently, the recombinant forms of aprotinin also became available; however, these variants are not clinically developed. With the additional pharmacologic knowledge, the application of this agent will be expanded for both medical and surgical indications. The anti-inflammatory components in aprotinin may be significantly higher than in other serine proteases, which are also listed in Table 8. However, additional studies are needed to compare the effect of aprotinin with that of these inhibitors.

Synthetic and recombinant agents such as ε-aminocaproic acid (EACA), tranexamic acid, and recombinant PAI are only useful in controlling fibrinolysis-mediated bleeding. However, their role as anti-inflammatory agents is not established. The pharmacologic profile of these agents as antifibrinolytic drugs also markedly differs from that of aprotinin. Thus, each of these agents should be used in individual indications at proper dosages and with well-defined approaches.

Heparin cofactor II and antithrombin III (AT-III) concentrates have been primarily developed for the control of thrombophilic conditions. While AT-III is now in clinical use globally, the development of heparin cofactor II is somewhat slow due to its weak antithrombin activity. Recombinant equivalents of both agents have also been produced; however, their clinical development is not evident at this time.

Antithrombin III has been used in disseminated intravascular coagulation (DIC) and the control of sepsis-induced hypercoagulable state. In these indications, it has been observed that this agent may have some anti-inflammatory properties; however, its role as an anti-inflammatory agent is not clearly established.

Heparin is one of the most widely used anticoagulants and has multiple sites of actions. Its anti-inflammatory actions have been known since its initial clinical use. However, the exact mechanism by which this agent produces anti-inflammatory effects was not fully understood until this time. Heparin is now known to produce a dose- and route-dependent release of TFPI. This inhibitor may have a strong anti-inflammatory effect that is primarily due to its polydomain antiprotease nature. The availability of recombinant TFPI has provided an opportunity to investigate this effect in the clinical setting. While the data are rather limited at this time, it appears that TFPI may play an important role in the control of inflammatory pathways at multiple points. Recombinant TFPI and its variants may, therefore, be useful as anti-inflammatory agents for various indications.

Many synthetic and recombinant antithrombin agents are being developed for various thrombotic and cardiovascular indications, including hirudin, hirulog, efegatran, and argatroban. These agents are capable of providing a specific inhibition of thrombin, but, unlike heparin, they do not produce any release of TFPI. No information on anti-inflammatory actions is available at this time. However, it is known that thrombin may contribute to the pathophysiology of inflammation. Furthermore, most of the thrombin inhibitors are being developed for various thrombotic and cardiovascular indications. Their use in sepsis- and cancer-mediated inflammatory conditions is rather limited. Thus, it appears that these synthetic inhibitors have a rather limited potential in the control of inflammatory disorders.

The agent DX 9065a represents a factor Xa inhibitor with weaker inhibitory actions towards such serine proteases as plasmin, activated protein C, and kallikreins. This agent is currently developed for various thrombotic indications. Relatively little is known about its anti-inflammatory effect. However, some of the nonspecific antiprotease actions may be contributory to its anti-inflammatory response. Studies to further investigate these actions are warranted.

It is quite clear from this discussion that while both synthetic and recombinant serine proteases may modulate the inflammatory process, information on their actions is rather limited. Furthermore, it is also not known whether these actions are primarily related to their antiprotease spectrum or to other properties that may modulate various cellular receptors. The pathophysiology of inflammation is rather complicated and involves both cellular and humoral components. An agent capable of producing anti-inflammatory action must, therefore, exhibit a strong effect on one or more of the key steps involved in this process. At the present time, only aprotinin and TFPI meet this criterion and their potential should be assessed in both monotherapeutic and polytherapeutic approaches.

SUMMARY

Several of the SERPINs produce varying degrees of inhibition of the inflammatory pathways by both direct and indirect mechanisms. Of these SERPINs, C1 esterase inhibitor, α_1-antitrypsin, α_2-macroglobulin, and TFPI produce sizeable anti-inflammatory actions. Protease activation processes resulting in the formation of kallikreins and fibrinolytic enzymes such as plasmin and plasminogen activators play an important role in the inflammatory response. Measurement of such markers as prekallikrein, bradykinin, anaphylotoxins, and some of the markers of fibrinolytic activation provides a useful means of evaluating the pathophysiologic activation of the inflammatory process and its modulation by SERPINs.

Aprotinin is a potent inhibitor of both plasmin and the kallikreins. In addition, aprotinin produces some direct effects on cellular sites. Aprotinin has been known to strongly inhibit the generation of bradykinin in both in vitro and in vivo experimental conditions. Thus, this agent represents a relatively strong anti-inflammatory substance.[9-12] The use of aprotinin during CPB not only reduces bleeding but may also inhibit various inflammatory processes. This is evident in clinical studies where the aprotinin treatment results in the inhibition of bradykinin generation and decreased circulating PMN elastase levels.

In contrast, aprotinin administration during cardiovascular surgery does not produce any major alterations in the neuropeptides such as substance P, neuropeptides Y, A, and CGRP. Since one of the functional domains of TFPI mimics aprotinin, these two agents may produce augmented inhibition of bradykinin formation and elastase release during cardiovascular surgery where the administration of large amounts of heparin results in up to a five-fold increase in TFPI release. Aprotinin is known to modulate the tissue factor-mediated activation of the coagulation system.[13] On the other hand, TFPI is known to inhibit thrombogenesis in vascular trauma as studied in animal models.[14] Thus, TFPI and aprotinin may also produce a mutually synergistic inhibition of tissue factor mediation of cellular and plasmatic activation processes. This modulation of the tissue factor may also contribute to the anti-inflammatory effects of these inhibitors.

Recombinant forms of aprotinin and TFPI thus represent two important agents that may play an important role in the control of inflammation. These agents warrant further clinical development in well-defined clinical trials addressing various inflammatory disorders.

References

1. Katunuma N, Kido H. Recent advances in research on tryptases and endogenous tryptase inhibitors. *Monogra Allergy* 1990;27:51-66.

2. Schoeffel U, Lausen M, Ruf G, von Specht BU, Freudenberg N. The overwhelming inflammatory response and the role of endotoxin in early sepsis. *Prog Clin Biol Res* 1989;308:371-376.

3. Knauer DJ, Thompson JA, Cunningham DD. Protease nexins: cell-secreted proteins that mediate the binding, internalization and degradation of regulatory serine proteases. *J Cell Physiol* 1983;117:385-396.

4. Broze GJ, Warren LP, Novotny WF, Higuchi DA, Girard JJ, Miletich JP. Lipoprotein-associated coagulation inhibitor that inhibits the factor VII tissue factor complex also inhibits factor Xa: insight into its possible mechanism of action. *Blood* 1988;71:335-343.

5. Hoppensteadt D, Walenga JM, Fasanella A, Jeske W, Fareed J. TFPI antigen levels in normal human volunteers after IV and SC administration of heparin and a low-molecular-weight heparin. *Thromb Res* 1994;77(2):175-185.

6 Hoppensteadt DA, Fasanella A, Fareed J. Effect of protamine on heparin releasable TFPI antigen levels in normal volunteers. *Thromb Res* 1995;79(3):325-330.

7. Jeske W, Hoppensteadt D, Klauser R, Kammereit A, Eckenberger P, Haas S, Wyld P, Fareed J: Effect of repeated aprosulate and enoxaparin administration on tissue factor pathway inhibitor antigen levels. *Blood Coag Fibrinol* 1995;6:119-124.

8. Fareed J, Callas D, Hoppensteadt D, Walenga J. Modulation of endothelium by heparin and related polyelectrolytes. In: Born GVR, Vane J, Welzel D, eds *The Endothelial Cell in Health and Diseases.* New York,NY: Shattauer Suttgart, pp 165-182.

9. Fareed J, Jeske W, Hoppensteadt D, Walenga JM, Pifarre R. Drug interactions with aprotinin. In: Pirarre R, ed. *Blood Conservation With Aprotinin,* Hanley & Belfus, Inc., Philadelphia, Pa: 1995: 215.

10. Fareed J, Hoppensteadt D, Koza MJ, Jeske W, Walenga JM, Pifarre R. Pharmacokinetics of aprotinin and its relevance to antifibrinolytic and other biologic effects. In: Pirarre R, ed. *Blood Conservation With Aprotinin,* Hanley & Belfus, Inc., Philadelphia, Pa: 1995: 131.

11. *Blood Conservation With Aprotinin.* Pifarre R. ed., Hanely & Belfus Inc' Philadelphia, Pa: 1995.

12. Westaby S. Aprotinin in perspective. *Ann Thorac Surg* 1993;55:1033-1041.

13. Van den Besselar AM, Dirven R, Bertina RM. Tissue factor-induced coagulation can be inhibited by aprotinin (Trasylol). *Thromb Haemost* 1993;69:298-299. Letter.

14. Khouri RK, Koudsi D, Fu K, Ornberg RL, Wun TC. Prevention of thrombosis by topical application of tissue factor pathway inhibitor in a rabbit model of vascular trauma. *Ann Plast Surg* 1993;30(5):398-404.

Fibrinolytic Activity During and After Surgery With Cardiopulmonary Bypass: Effects of Aprotinin

He Lu, MD, Claudine Soria, PhD, Charles Du Buit, MD,
Pierre Commin, MD, Bernard Touchot, MD,
Bernard Chollet, MD, Jeannette Soria, PhD

Intraoperative and postoperative blood loss during open heart surgery with cardiopulmonary bypass (CPB) can be reduced by 50% with aprotinin therapy.[1-4] To explore the mechanism of this effect we conducted a number of studies to investigate the action of aprotinin on coagulation and fibrinolysis during and after CPB.

OVERVIEW OF FIBRINOLYSIS

Fibrinolysis is initiated by the conversion of the inactive zymogen plasminogen to the protease plasmin that degrades fibrin into soluble fibrin degradation products (FbDP). The two main plasminogen activators are tissue-type plasminogen activator (t-PA) and urinary-type plasminogen activator (u-PA), or urokinase (UK). Tissue plasminogen activator, which has the most potent action to initiate thrombolysis, is secreted in an active form from endothelial cells, whereas u-PA exists in blood as an inactive zymogen in single-chain form (scu-PA or pro-urokinase) and can be converted to the active two-chain form (urokinase) by trace amounts of plasmin or kallikrein, usually near the surface of the thrombus.

The action of t-PA is greatly enhanced in the presence of fibrin due to the formation of a ternary fibrin/t-PA/plasminogen complex. This ensures that plasmin is restricted to within the thrombus and very little is free in the circulation. In addition, free plasmin is immediately inactivated in plasma by the fast inhibitor α_2-antiplasmin. The plasmin degrades fibrin into FbDP that contain the D-dimer moiety. Aprotinin can inhibit plasmin generated within the fibrin clot by binding to the active serine enzymatic site.[5]

The activity of plasminogen activators is regulated by a series of inhibitors, the most important of which in plasma is the plasminogen activator inhibitor type 1 (PAI-1).

Action of Plasmin on Platelets

Platelets initiate hemostasis by adhering to subendothelial surfaces after blood vessels have been damaged. This adhesion is mediated by the interaction of platelet glycoprotein (GP) complex GP1b/GPIX with the subendothelium-bound von Willebrand factor (vWF).[6] Plasmin will affect platelet function by inducing either platelet activation or inhibition, depending on the dose and temperature, and by reducing the interaction between platelet GPIb and vWF.[7-10] Fibrinolysis is known to be activated during CPB, and the effects of plasmin on platelet function might therefore be expected to occur in vivo during open heart surgery.[11]

The bulk of GPIb lies exterior to the platelet surface and is present in the intact membrane as a complex with GPIX. This complex is linked to actin filaments of the submembrane cytoskeletal network indirectly through actin-binding protein.[12] Until recently, it was thought that the cleavage of GPIb by plasmin was the major cause of the reduction of vWF binding to platelets, since a fragment of GPIb called glycocalicin has been detected in the supernatant of platelet suspension after incubation with high concentrations of plasmin.[9] In contrast, we recently demonstrated, using electron microscopy and an immunogold-staining technique for GPIb, that plasmin at low concentrations induces platelet structural changes, including shape change, pseudopod formation, centralization of platelet granules, and translocation of platelet GPIb from the plasma membrane into the surface-connected canalicular system without any evident degranulation.[7,13] Neutralization of plasmin by its inhibitor, aprotinin, reversed this translocation and restored a normal amount of GPIb on the platelet surface and also restored normal platelet adhesive function.[14]

Platelet adhesion is commonly assessed in vitro using ristocetin to induce agglutination. Clinically, patients undergoing open heart surgery with CPB show a plasmin-related anomaly in ristocetin-induced platelet agglutination.[15] The action of aprotinin seen with electron microscopy to reverse translocation of GPIb on the platelet surface was supported by the results of the platelet functional agglutination tests with ristocetin which is a marker of vWF dependent-platelet adhesiveness (Fig 1). Aprotinin induced a progressive recovery of the capacity of platelets to agglutinate with ristocetin.

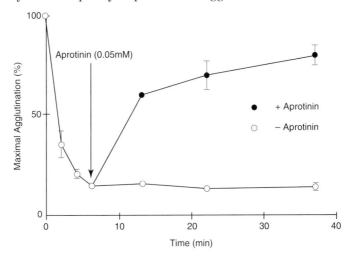

Fig 1. Ristocetin-induced platelet agglutination of plasmin-treated platelets before and after addition of aprotinin. Mean ± SE for six donors. (Reproduced with permission from *European Journal of Clinical Investigation* 1993;23:788.)

Regulation of the Fibrinolytic System by PAI-1

An imbalance in the perioperative levels of PAI-1 in patients undergoing major surgery may result in posttraumatic hemorrhage (decreased activity) or be associated with a thrombotic risk (increased activity). Significant increases in PAI-1 have been shown to occur in patients postoperatively.[16] Many inflammatory mediators can stimulate release of PAI-1 from endothelial cells (interleukin-1, tumor necrosis factor, lipopolysaccharide, TGF beta), although the stimulus for the postoperative increase in PAI-1 has not been identified. The action of one or more mediators in plasma is supported by the demonstration in vitro of a three-fold increase in the ability of postoperative plasma compared with preoperative plasma to stimulate PAI-1 release from endothelial cells in culture. Increased PAI-1 secretion peaks between postoperative day 1 and 2 and is temporally associated with a fall in D-dimer, a degradation product of fibrin indicating a hypofibrinolytic state in patients at this time.[17] This, together with hypercoagulability from increased expression of tissue factor, may predispose the patient towards a thrombotic state in the immediate postoperative period.

Other studies have shown elevated PAI-1 levels to be associated with early atherosclerosis and recurrence of myocardial infarction.[18,19]

The association between increased PAI-1 levels and increased risk of deep-vein thrombosis and arterial injury may be a direct consequence of fibrin deposition related to imbalance between plasminogen activator and plasminogen activator inhibitor. However, this has not been proved, and the increased secretion of PAI-1 may merely be a marker of endothelial dysfunction, possibly as a consequence of cytokine-induced vessel injury.

APROTININ'S ACTIONS ON PERIOPERATIVE FIBRINOLYSIS AND COAGULATION

Open heart surgery with CPB is associated with abnormal blood loss and excessive blood transfusion.[20,21] Aprotinin, a potent inhibitor of plasmin and kallikrein, is widely accepted as effective therapy for this patient population. Our clinical research has been directed towards elucidating the mechanism by which aprotinin can substantially reduce blood loss and the need for blood and blood-product replacement and towards investigating the possibility that this agent's antifibrinolytic action may increase the risk of thrombotic complications both during surgery and in the postoperative period.

Plasma levels of thrombin-induced modified antithrombin III (ATM) were measured as a marker of activation of coagulation with thrombin generation, and t-PA, PAI-1, and D-dimer activity measured as fibrinolytic system markers. Platelet adhesive function was evaluated on washed platelets with ristocetin-induced agglutination. Patients randomized to the aprotinin group received the high-dose regimen, according to Royston.[22] This dosage protocol will achieve plasma levels > 4μm and effectively inhibit plasmin and kallikrein. Heparin administration was adjusted to maintain plasma levels above 4 IU/mL.

Study 1: Coagulation and Fibrinolysis During Surgery[15]

This study was conducted during the perioperative period and aimed to investigate the mechanism of the effective and significant reduction in bleeding achieved with aprotinin administration.

Patients were randomly allocated to receive aprotinin or a placebo (10 patients per group). Blood samples were collected from each patient at four different time points during the operation. The first sample (T1) was drawn before anesthesia and the administration of aprotinin or placebo. The second sample (T2) was drawn 30 minutes after the start of CPB during hypothermia. The third sample (T3) was drawn after cross-clamp removal during rewarming, and the fourth sample (T4), 10 minutes after heparin reversal with protamine.

Despite the very high concentration of heparin used to avoid clot formation during bypass, a low level of fibrin formation still occurred and underwent degradation in the placebo group as shown by the increase in D-dimer, whereas the aprotinin-treated group had lower levels of D-dimer. There was a progressive increase in the plasma concentration of D-dimer (DDE) complexes in the placebo group during surgery. Aprotinin effectively inhibited the generation of DDE complexes during CPB, although a slight elevation was noticed at the end of the operation in the aprotinin group (Fig 2).

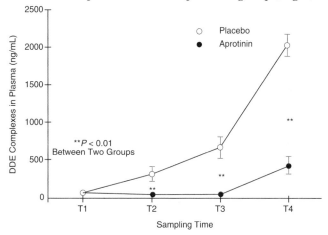

Fig 2. Plasma level of D-dimer (DDE) complexes. Mean ± SE. (Reproduced with permission from *Thrombosis and Hemostasis* 1991;66:635.)

A more important finding was the protective effect of aprotinin in maintaining normal platelet adhesiveness. The placebo group showed a continuous decrease in platelet ristocetin-induced agglutination during CPB (Fig 3). As mentioned previously, this decreased agglutination reflects impaired platelet adhesion due to internalization of platelet GPIb receptors on the plasma membrane as a result of low levels of plasmin activity in the plasma. In contrast, ristocetin-induced agglutination was unaffected in samples from aprotinin-treated patients. The constant generation of thrombin during CPB was shown by elevated levels of ATM in both groups, although levels in the aprotinin-treated group were significantly lower at the end of CPB (Fig 4).

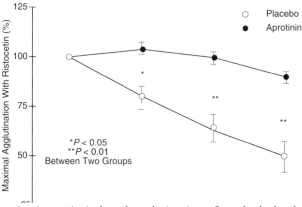

Fig 3. Changes in ristocetin-induced agglutination of washed platelets. The results of samples T2-T4 were calculated as a percentage of the maximal agglutination of sample T1. (Reproduced with permission from *Thrombosis and Hemostasis* 1991;66:634.)

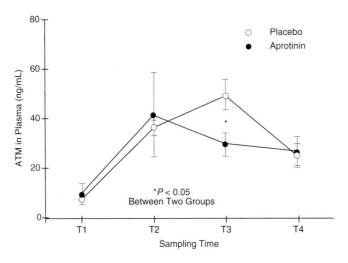

Fig 4. Plasma level of modified antithrombin III (ATM). Mean ± SE. (Reproduced with permission from *Thrombosis and Hemostasis* 1991;66:635.)

The differences found between the placebo- and aprotinin-treated patients could be due to an antikallikrein action of aprotinin, since kallikrein potentiates the contact-phase activation of coagulation that occurs within the extracorporeal circuit.

Study 2: Coagulation and Fibrinolysis After Surgery[17]

This study was undertaken to evaluate the effects of aprotinin administration on in vivo thrombolysis both during and after CPB, with emphasis on the duration and extent of the antifibrinolytic action of aprotinin during the postoperative period.

Patients were randomly allocated to receive aprotinin (16 patients) or a placebo (14 patients). Blood samples were collected from each patient at four different time points during the operation. The first sample was drawn before anesthesia and the administration of aprotinin or placebo (T1). The second sample (D0) was drawn 2 hours after the end of surgery. Samples D1 to D11 are subsequent postoperative days.

As in Study 1, high levels of fibrinolytic activity were evidenced during the surgery, as judged by high levels of FbDP in the placebo group (Fig 5), and this activity was inhibited by aprotinin. During the first postoperative day, there was a rapid decrease in FbDP levels in the placebo group, while levels in the aprotinin group remained consistently low. The same nadir for the two groups was reached by the second postoperative day, and levels then started to increase up to the ninth postoperative day in an identical manner for the two groups. A significant increase in both t-PA and PAI-1 levels was found at D0 (Figs 6 and 7). There were no significant differences in t-PA levels between both groups, with levels declining immediately after surgery. In contrast to the rapid decline in t-PA levels, PAI-1 levels did not change between D0 and D1 in the aprotinin group, whereas in the placebo group, the PAI-1 level showed a further increase. The difference between the level of PAI-1 24 hours after surgery and the preoperative level of PAI-1 was significantly higher in the placebo group. After day 1, t-PA continued to decrease and PAI-1 began to decrease steadily.

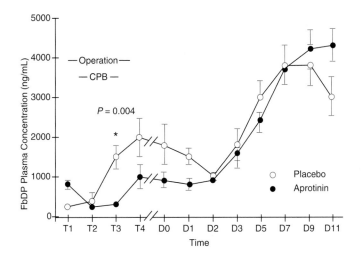

Fig 5. Plasma levels of fibrin degradation products (FbDP) during and after surgery. Mean ± SE. (Reproduced with permission from *Thrombosis and Hemostasis* 1994;72:440.)

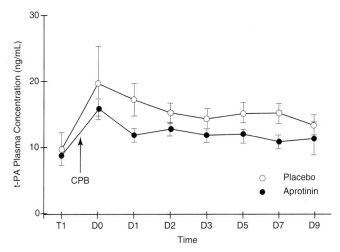

Fig 6. Plasma levels of tissue-type plasminogen activator (t-PA) before and after surgery. Mean ± SE. (Reproduced with permission from *Thrombosis and Hemostasis* 1994;72:440.)

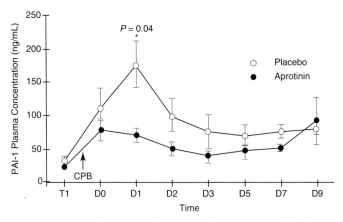

Fig 7. Plasma levels of plasminogen activator inhibitor type 1 (PAI-1) before and after surgery. Mean ± SE. CPB, Cardiopulmonary bypass. (Reproduced with permission from *Thrombosis and Hemostasis* 1994;72:441.)

However, it still remains to be clarified whether the high postoperative PAI-1 levels predispose to an early thrombotic risk and whether it is possible to set a threshold of postoperative PAI-1 values to allow the identification of patients at greater risk of postoperative thrombotic events. Plasminogen activator inhibitor type 1 is also considered to be a fast reactant protein, so that the important increase noted in the placebo group may reflect a general response to multiple trauma due to activation of white blood cells and complement factors responsible for endothelial cell damage. In this case, the lower level of PAI-1 in the aprotinin group may result from the reduced inflammatory reaction in these patients. At present, it is unclear whether the reduction in PAI-1 results from the antiplasmin or the antikallikrein activity of aprotinin, or both. Whatever the mechanism involved, aprotinin showed a new beneficial effect in open heart surgery. However, due to the small size of this study, a number of questions remain to be determined in further clinical studies in larger groups of patients.

As seen in Study 1, activation of blood coagulation, as shown by ATM levels, occurred in both groups during surgery but to a lesser extent in aprotinin-treated patients. Postoperatively, the plasma levels of ATM decreased to baseline values by the first postoperative day and remained at this level in both groups, with no significant differences between the groups.

SUMMARY

The results of our studies show an important release of t-PA and PAI-1-induced by open heart surgery with CPB. However, t-PA release was quickly turned off after surgery (as indicated by an immediate decrease after surgery), while PAI-1 release was prolonged. The peak level of PAI-1 was found at 24 hours after surgery in the placebo group. This high PAI-1 level may have contributed to postoperative hemostasis by preventing premature breakdown of fibrin clots, since FbDP levels were low for the first 48 hours in these patients. The PAI-1 levels in the aprotinin group during the first postoperative day were much lower than those in the placebo group. The important increase in PAI-1 can explain the postoperative decrease in D-dimers in the first 2 postoperative days in the placebo group. There was no obvious effect of aprotinin on fibrinolysis 48 hours after CPB, indicating that intraoperative administration of aprotinin did not result in a delayed degradation of fibrin after surgery.

REFERENCES

1. Royston D. High-dose aprotinin therapy: a review of the first five years' experience. *J Cardiothorac Vasc Anesth* 1992;6:76-100.

2. Bidstrup BP, Royston D, Sapsford RN, Taylor KM. Reduction in blood loss and blood use after cardiopulmonary bypass with high dose aprotinin (Trasylol). *J Thorac Cardiovasc Surg* 1989;97:364-372.

3. Lemmer J Jr, Stanford W, Bonney SL, et al. Aprotinin for coronary bypass operations: efficacy, safety, and influence on early saphenous vein graft patency. A multicenter, randomized, double-blind, placebo-controlled study. *J Thorac Cardiovasc Surg* 1994;107:543-551.

4. Dietrich W, Spannagl M, Jochum M, et al. Influence of high-dose aprotinin treatment on blood loss and coagulation patterns in patients undergoing myocardial revascularization. *Anesthesiology* 1990;73:1119-1126. Comments.

5. Verstraete M. Clinical application of inhibitors of fibrinolysis. *Drugs* 1985;29:236-261.

6. George J, Nurden A, Phillips D. Molecular defects in interactions of platelets with the vessel wall. *N Engl J Med* 1984;311:1084-1098.

7. Lu H, Soria C, Cramer E, et al. Temperature dependence of plasmin activation or inhibition of human platelet. *Blood* 1991;77:996-1005.

8. Lu H, Soria C, Li H, et al. Role of active center and lysine binding sites of plasmin in plasmin-induced platelet activation. *Thromb Haemost* 1991;65:67-72.

9. Adelman B, Michelson A, Loscalzo J, Greenberg J, Handin R. Plasmin effect on platelet glycoprotein 1b-von Willebrand factor interactions. *Blood* 1985;65:32-40.

10. Michelson A, Bernard M. Plasmin-induced redistribution of platelet glycoprotein 1b. *Blood* 1990;76:2005-2010.

11. Tanaka K, Morimoto T, Yada I, Kusagawa M, Degushi K. Physiologic role of enhanced fibrinolytic activity during cardiopulmonary bypass in open heart surgery. *Trans ASAIO* 1987;33:505-509.

12. Okita J, Pidard D, Newman P, Montgomery R, Kunicki T. On the association of glycoprotein 1b and actin-binding protein in human platelets. *J Cell Biol* 1985;100:317-321.

13. Cramer E, Lu H, Caen J, Soria C, Tanza D. Differential redistribution of glycoprotein Ib and IIb-IIIa after plasmin stimulation. *Blood* 1991;77:694-699.

14. Lu H, Soria C, Soria J, et al. Reversible translocation of glycoprotein Ib in plasmin-treated platelets: consequences for platelet function. *Eur J Clin Invest* 1993;23:785-793.

15. Lu H, Soria C, Commin PL, et al. Hemostasis in patients undergoing extracorporeal circulation: the effect of aprotinin (Trasylol). *Thromb Haemost* 1991;66:633-637.

16. Paramo J, Rifon J, Llorens R, Casares J, Paloma M, Rocha E. Intra- and postoperative fibrinolysis in patients undergoing cardiopulmonary bypass. *Haemostasis* 1991;21:58-64.

17. Lu H, Du-Buit C, Soria J, et al. Postoperative hemostasis and fibrinolysis in patients undergoing cardiopulmonary bypass with or without aprotinin therapy. *Thromb Haemost* 1994;72:438-443.

18. Meade TW, Ruddock V, Stirling Y, Chakrabarti R, Miller GJ. Fibrinolytic activity, clotting factors, and long-term incidence of ischaemic heart disease in the Northwick Park Heart Study. *Lancet.* 1993;342:1076-1079. Comments.

19. Hamsten A, de Faire U, Walldius G, et al. Plasminogen activator inhibitor in plasma: risk factor for recurrent myocardial infarction. *Lancet* 1987;2:3-9 .

20. Bick R. Hemostasis defects associated with cardiac surgery, prosthetic devices, and other extracorporeal circuits. *Semin Thromb Hemost* 1985;11:249-280.

21. Hunt B. Modifying perioperative blood loss. *Blood Rev* 1991;5:168-176.

22. Royston D, Bidstrup BP, Taylor KM, Sapsford RN. Effect of aprotinin on need for blood transfusion after repeat open-heart surgery. *Lancet* 1987;2:1289-1291.

Using Pharmacologic Agents in Combination

Jeanine M. Walenga, PhD, FACA, Mark R. Terrell, MD, Roque Pifarré, MD

Surgical patients are often administered an array of drugs that may include antimicrobial, anti-inflammatory, analgesic, and antihypertensive agents, as well as antithrombotic and other specific cardiac agents. Each drug will have both known and unknown effects, and each could have multiple sites of action. A clinically important situation may arise in these patients from drug-drug interactions, some of which are documented but others we may not be aware of, particularly in the case of newly available drugs. Interaction between drugs may be beneficial to the patient synergistically or additively; on the other hand, agents in combination may produce unwanted side effects.

Alteration of the hemostatic balance in cardiac surgical patients exposed to numerous drugs is an important example of drug interactions. Of particular relevance are drugs that potentiate or inhibit the anticoagulant actions of heparin; activate or inhibit the fibrinolytic system, the kallikrein system; inhibit platelet function; and modulate endothelial cell function. Volume expansion and altered blood viscosity can alter hemostasis. Many substances and drugs of widely differing modes of action can influence hemostasis (Table 1).[1]

Table 1. Drugs and Other Substances That Interact With the Hemostatic System

Drug/Substance	Fibrinolysis	Platelet Function	Coagulation
Antineoplastic drugs	+	+	+
Autonomic drugs	+	+	ND
Steroids	+	+	ND
Hormones	+	+	+
Antibiotics	+	+	-
Analgesics	ND	+	-
Antipsychotics	ND	+	ND
B-Blockers	+	+	ND
Diuretics	ND	+	-
Lipid-lowering agents	±	+	ND
Anticonvulsants	ND	ND	ND
Antacids	ND	ND	-
Antihistamines	±	+	-
Food	±	+	+
Caffeine	±	+	-
Alcohol	+	+	-

ND, not determined.

EFFECTS OF HEPARIN ON HEMOSTASIS

The study of drug interactions is made more difficult in that drugs do not necessarily have one mechanism of action. Drugs can have other actions related or unrelated to their target mechanism, actions known or unknown.

Heparin is a drug administered for its known action as an anticoagulant, but which in itself has additional actions on the hemostatic balance of the patient. Heparin complexed to antithrombin III (AT-III) inhibits factors Xa and IIa. However, this complex can also inhibit factors IXa, XIIa, and XIa to produce its anticoagulant effect. Heparin and related glycosaminoglycans are bound to the endothelial cell surface of blood vessels and play a key role in maintaining vascular integrity.[2] Vascular smooth-muscle cells (SMC), growth factors, and possibly cytokines are affected by heparin.[3,4] Heparin is neutralized by platelet factor 4 and neutrophil lactoferrin.[5,6] It was recently discovered that heparin releases tissue factor pathway inhibitor (TFPI), a natural inhibitor of factor VIIa/factor Xa.[7]

Low-molecular-weight heparin (LMWH) is now considered the drug of choice for prophylaxis against deep-vein thrombosis (DVT) in postoperative patients undergoing both general and orthopedic surgical procedures. A recent study carried out at Loyola University Medical Center investigated the role of TFPI in mediating the antithrombotic activity of LMWH.[8] Plasma levels of TFPI were measured in a group of postorthopedic surgery patients given daily subcutaneous injections of LMWH and in a group of patients given a placebo. In the placebo group (n = 25), the plasma TFPI levels were slightly elevated immediately after surgery but returned to their baseline value by the fifth postoperative day. In contrast, in the LMWH group (n = 34), the plasma levels of TFPI increased significantly and remained elevated for up to 7 days after surgery. However, the TFPI levels in both groups showed wide patient-to-patient variability.

Similar results were found in patients at Loyola undergoing percutaneous transluminal coronary angioplasty (PTCA) and during surgery with cardiopulmonary bypass (CPB [Fig 1]). Both procedures require anticoagulation of the patient with heparin, which is associated with a very significant dose-dependent increase in TFPI release. This previously unknown release of TFPI associated with heparin contributes to the anticoagulant effect of this drug and may account for poor response to heparinization in some patients.

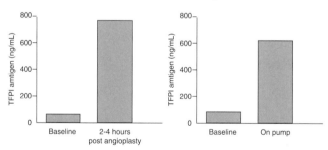

Fig 1. A, Tissue factor pathway inhibitor (TFPI) levels in patients undergoing angioplasty are greatly enhanced due to heparin. TFPI levels are related to heparin dose and return to normal by 24 hours after heparin administration. B, Tissue factor pathway inhibitor (TFPI) levels in cardiopulmonary bypass (CPB) patients are greatly enhanced due to heparin. After protamine administration, TFPI levels return to normal.

In patients undergoing therapy for thrombotic events a combination of drugs may be used to target specific areas for treatment. Patients may be receiving antiplatelet agents, oral or intravenous anticoagulants, and thrombolytic drugs. The benefits of multiple targets for treatment may also incur the risk of an enhanced bleeding side effect. This is evidenced from the recent Global Use of strategies to Open Occluded Coronary Arteries (GUSTO IIa); Hirudin for Improvement of Thrombolysis (HITIII); and Thrombolysis and Thrombin Inhibition in Myocardial Infarction (TIMI9A) clinical trials in which aspirin was used in combination with hirudin and thrombolytic therapy. A trend of enhanced hemorrhagic stroke or nonintracranial hemorrhage was found in comparison with heparin in all groups.[9-11]

For the patient undergoing cardiac surgery, the perioperative period comprises numerous physical interventions and traumas, drug administration (anesthetics, anticoagulants, and protamine in particular), and other invasive treatments (eg, cardioplegia, hemodilution, hypothermia, CPB, foreign-material implants), causing activation of plasma proteins and platelets, which further contributes to hemostatic modulation. Thus, the surgical patient is at an enhanced risk of perioperative blood loss from several factors, including combined drug effects.

BLOOD PRESERVATION IN CARDIAC SURGERY

Patients undergoing cardiac surgery with CPB are at increased risk of perioperative blood loss requiring blood and blood-product transfusion. Dr Roque Pifarré at Loyola has taken a particular interest in the possible causes of this problem and has developed a blood-conservation program that has reduced perioperative blood loss at our institution to levels lower than the national average.[12] The protocol involves: (1) securing a thorough patient history and physical examination preoperatively to identify patients at increased risk of perioperative bleeding either because of inherited or acquired disease associated with hemostatic disorders or because of concomitant drug therapy, eg, aspirin; (2) encouraging patients to predonate autologous blood; (3) using cell salvage to wash and reinfuse blood lost from the surgical site; (4) monitoring activated clotting time (ACT) during surgery to ensure adequate heparin levels (in the early years of cardiac surgery when monitoring was not available, patients were often given too much heparin to ensure adequate anticoagulation, thus increasing postoperative bleeding); and (5) monitoring protamine sulfate reversal of heparinization and giving protamine as a split dose— two-thirds at the time of separation from bypass and the remaining third when all the autologous and salvaged blood has been reinfused.

This protocol reduced the perioperative blood loss from approximately 850 mL/24h to 500 mL/24h when ACT monitoring was introduced. Monitoring the protamine dosage and timing its administration further reduced the average blood loss to between 300 mL and 400 mL for a 24-hour perioperative period.[13]

BLEEDING ASSOCIATED WITH CPB SURGERY

Despite meticulous surgical technique and a well adhered to blood-conservation program, some patients still have excessive bleeding associated with CPB. Functional platelet defects, induced either by the extracorporeal circuit or by drug administration, are the most common cause of postoperative bleeding.[14] The fibrinolytic components of the hemostatic system are activated during CPB. In some patients, hyperfibrinolysis may become excessive and uncompensated and in rare cases lead to disseminated intravascular coagulopathy (DIC).[15] Thrombocytopenia may result in defective hemostasis, and incorrect heparin/protamine dosage or heparin rebound are all possible, although not common reasons for increased perioperative bleeding.

Managing Excessive Bleeding

To counteract adverse bleeding, cryoprecipitate, platelet concentrates, desmopressin acetate, an arginine vasopressin derivative that increases factor VIII levels, and ε-aminocaproic acid (to reverse excess fibrinolysis) have been in use for years. More recently, aprotinin was proved to have a clinically significant effect in reducing postoperative blood loss after a variety of surgical procedures; in particular, a large number of clinical trials have shown it to have consistent efficacy in improving hemostasis after cardiac surgery.[16-18] A comparative study at Loyola of aprotinin administration in combination with the institution's blood-conservation protocol decreased the 24-hour blood loss from an average of 600 mL to 300 mL. Similar efficacy was seen when results from the published literature were compared. These showed a reduction from 1200 mL/24-h period without aprotinin to approximately 700 mL with aprotinin therapy. Interestingly, the amount of bleeding postoperatively at Loyola is significantly less than the average nationwide published figures.

Aprotinin is a nonspecific serine protease inhibitor that inhibits trypsin, chymotrypsin, kallikrein, plasmin, thrombin, and protein C by reversibly binding to these enzymes.[19-21] Tissue factor and neutrophil elastase may also be inhibited by aprotinin.[22] Besides its effects on fibrinolysis and coagulation, aprotinin interacts with leukocytes, endothelial cells, and platelets.[23] It has been speculated, based on its structure, that aprotinin may act as a nitric oxide donor, thereby modulating cellular responses (personal communication). The basic mechanism of aprotinin in reducing postoperative blood loss is complex and not clearly defined. Inhibition of the contact/coagulation system (via kallikrein inhibition), the attenuation of fibrinolytic activation to improve clot stability, coupled with a platelet 'protective' effect (via plasmin inhibition) may all contribute to a greater or lesser extent to the in vivo action of aprotinin in improving hemostasis.[24-27]

Antifibrinolytic Activity of Aprotinin

The ability of aprotinin to attenuate the fibrinolytic activation associated with CPB was assessed in a recent study at Loyola. These data were collected as part of a multicenter randomized, double-blind, placebo-controlled trial to determine the optimal dosing regimen for efficacy (reduction of postoperative blood loss) and safety in patients undergoing repeat myocardial revascularization surgery.[28] Patients were administered one of three doses of aprotinin or placebo and blood samples collected pre-, intra-, and postoperatively for assay of fibrinolytic parameters to determine the association of the fibrinolytic state with postsurgical bleeding.[29] The four treatment arms are shown in Table 2. Treatment was begun after induction of anesthesia and continued until the patient was transferred to the intensive care unit.

Table 2. Multicenter Aprotinin Treatment Arms

	Loading Dose	Continuous Infusion Dose	CPB Prime Dose
Group I (n = 11) (High-dose 4.5 mu)	Aprotinin 280 mg	Aprotinin 70 mg/h	Aprotinin 280 mg
Group II (n = 11) (Low-dose 2.25 mu)	Aprotinin 140 mg + placebo	Aprotinin 35 mg/h + placebo	Aprotinin 140 mg + placebo
Group III (n = 7) (2 mu, pump prime)	Placebo	Placebo	Aprotinin 280 mg
Placebo (n = 7)	Placebo	Placebo	Placebo

CPB, cardiopulmonary bypass; mu, million units.

Fibrin degradation products (FDP) were significantly increased postoperatively in the placebo group (Fig 2). Levels fell 24 hours after surgery, although not to within the normal range. The two higher-dose aprotinin groups revealed only a slight postoperative rise, whereas the lowest-dose aprotinin group (pump prime only) had a similar response to the placebo group, with significantly elevated levels postoperatively. Tissue plasminogen activator (t-PA) antigen showed a slight decrease in all aprotinin groups on the pump, with an increase above baseline levels postoperatively (Fig 3). Levels at 24 hours were near preoperative levels, although elevated above the normal range. In contrast, in the placebo group the postoperative elevation in t-PA continued to increase through the next 24 hours. The inhibitor to t-PA, plasminogen activator inhibitor type 1 (PAI-1) antigen showed a slight on-pump decrease in all groups, followed by a postoperative increase that was more marked in the placebo and lowest-dose aprotinin groups (Fig 4). At 24 hours, a return towards preoperative levels occurred only in the aprotinin groups; levels in the placebo group remained elevated.

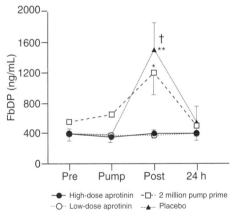

Fig 2. Fibrin degradation products (FbDP). Blood samples were collected from redo-CABG patients preoperatively prior to aprotinin administration, after 30 minutes on-pump, immediately after administration of protamine (post-pump), and 24 hours after surgery. The mean level of FbDPs (± SEM) is depicted for each aprotinin/placebo treatment group. The single asterisk (*) indicates $P < 0.05$ and the double asterisk (**), $P < 0.01$ versus the high-dose aprotinin value; the dagger (†) indicates $P < 0.01$ versus the preoperative value. (Reprinted with permission from Pa, Pifarré R, ed. *Blood Conservation with Aprotinin*. Philadephia, Pa: Hanley & Belfus;1995:185-197.)

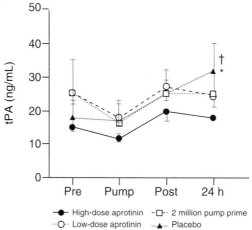

Fig 3. Tissue plasminogen activator (t-PA). Blood samples were collected from redo-CABG patients preoperatively prior to aprotinin administration, after 30 minutes on-pump, immediately after administration of protamine (post-pump), and 24 hours after surgery. The mean level of t-PA (± SEM) is depicted for each aprotinin/placebo treatment group. The asterisk (*) indicates $P < 0.05$ versus the high-dose aprotinin value; the dagger (†) indicates $P < 0.05$ versus the on-pump value. (Reprinted with permission from Pa, Pifarré R, ed. *Blood Conservation with Aprotinin*. Philadephia, Pa: Hanley & Belfus;1995:103-129.)

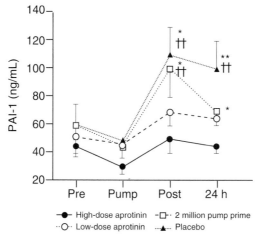

Fig 4. Plasminogen activator inhibitor (PAI-1).Blood samples were collected from redo-CABG patients preoperatively prior to aprotinin administration, after 30 minutes on-pump, immediately after administration of protamine (post-pump), and 24 hours after surgery. The mean level of PAI-1 (± SEM) is depicted for each aprotinin/placebo treatment group. The single asterisk (*) indicates $P < 0.05$ and the double asterisk (**) , $P < 0.01$ versus the high-dose aprotinin value; the double dagger (††) indicates $P < 0.01$ versus the on-pump value. (Reprinted with permission from Pa, Pifarré R, ed. *Blood Conservation with Aprotinin*. Philadephia, Pa: Hanley & Belfus;1995:103-129.)

This study revealed that fibrinolysis is enhanced during surgery with CPB. With aprotinin at the high dose, fibrinolysis is significantly reduced, with less t-PA and probably more active PAI-1 as well as other fibrinolytic inhibitors than in the nontreated placebo group. Other findings were observed with the coagulation (decreased thrombin generation) and platelet systems (decreased platelet activation), but no factor appeared important enough to be the primary mechanism by which aprotinin reduced postoperative blood loss.

The same study from Loyola showed that despite heparinization, there was still generation of thrombin during the bypass period, as evidenced by an increase in the thrombin-antithrombin III (TAT) complexes in the plasma (Fig 5). Aprotinin causes a dose-dependent reduction in the levels of TAT complexes, confirming the moderate anticoagulant effect of aprotinin reported in the literature,[30,31] and also demonstrating no procoagulant effect by aprotinin in these patients.

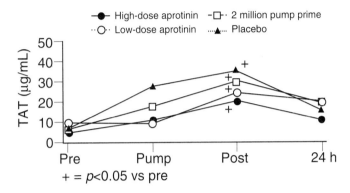

Fig 5. Thrombin-antithrombin (TAT) complex. Blood samples were collected from redo-CABG patients preoperatively prior to aprotinin administration, after 30 minutes on-pump, immediately after administration of protamine (post-pump), and 24 hours after surgery. The mean level of TAT (± SEM) is depicted for each aprotinin/placebo treatment group. The dagger (†) indicates $p < 0.05$ versus the pre-pump value.

Platelet Function and Aprotinin

Platelet activation and the release of α-granule contents are associated with the appearance on the platelet surface of the α-granule membrane protein (GMP-140), designated CD62 and also known as P-selectin. This glycoprotein is responsible for the adhesion of platelets to white cells. Using flow cytometry techniques in our laboratory at Loyola has allowed us to investigate CD62 expression on platelets sampled from patients undergoing CPB and receiving aprotinin therapy.[32] The results showed that throughout the perioperative period, circulating platelets from patients receiving aprotinin showed less autoactivation (no platelet agonist added to the test system) than those from control patients during CPB (Fig 6), as measured by expression of CD62 (implying platelet activation with α-granule release). If the platelets were stimulated with ristocetin (GPIb-mediated adhesion), the aprotinin-treated platelets were capable of expressing a significantly greater activation response. This was not the case for platelets sampled from patients not treated with aprotinin, which showed that only a decreased platelet activation response could be generated postoperatively, presumably because the platelets were spent during surgery. These data imply that aprotinin is able to minimize platelet activation during surgery and that the platelets have enhanced ability for adhesion postoperatively. These observations were more apparent for platelet-leukocyte than for platelet-platelet interactions.

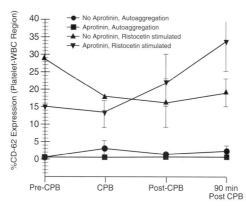

Fig 6. P-selectin (CD62) expression on platelets obtained from CPB patients undergoing surgery with and without aprotinin treatment. Blood samples were collected from redo-CABG patients preoperatively prior to aprotinin administration, after 30 minutes on-pump, immediately after administration of protamine (post-pump), and 90 minutes after surgery. The mean level of P-selectin (± SEM) is depicted for both aprotinin and placebo treatment groups. Autoactivation reflects circulating platelet activity (no agonist added to test system). Platelet response following ristocetin activation is also shown. Results are obtained from the flow cytometric analysis of the region threshold gated on platelet-leukocyte interaction.

Effects of Aprotinin on Anticoagulant Monitoring

Monitoring anticoagulation during CPB is very important, particularly if aprotinin is being used as part of a blood-conservation program. Most institutions perform routine monitoring of adequate heparin levels by measuring ACT.[33] Confusion has resulted from the finding that the celite - ACT is prolonged in the presence of aprotinin. Figure 7 shows data from our own institution, with values for aprotinin-treated patients exceeding 500 seconds in blood taken 10 minutes after heparin administration.[34] Adequate anticoagulation with heparin during CPB is achieved if the ACT is maintained at ≥ 400 seconds.[35] It was erroneously suggested that aprotinin provided additional anticoagulant effects during CPB and that heparin doses could be reduced.[36,37] A clinical study used the celite - ACT > 400 seconds as a minimum level of anticoagulation.[38] This trial showed a possible increase in thrombotic complications after patients undergoing repeat coronary artery bypass were treated with aprotinin, raising the question of whether aprotinin could be prothrombotic. The results of a multicenter randomized trial showed no such complications and suggest that the complications reported might have resulted from inadequate heparinization due to the belief that aprotinin decreased heparin requirements (Fig 5).[28]

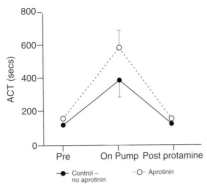

Fig 7. Effect of full-dose aprotinin supplementation on the celite activated clotting time during cardiopulmonary bypass with heparin. Results are mean ± standard deviation.(Reprinted with permission from *Ann Thor Surg* 93;55;662-666.)

We have shown that aprotinin has no effects on the other aspects of the coagulation profile (prothrombin time, thrombin time), demonstrating that the anticoagulant effect of aprotinin observed by ACT is not heparin-like.[34] It has been suggested that if aprotinin is used, the celite - ACT should be maintained at >750 seconds[39,40] or kaolin, which is unaffected by aprotinin, should be used as an alternative activator of clotting.[41]

Aprotinin and Alternative Anticoagulants

Alternative anticoagulants for use during CPB are undergoing clinical trials. We have evaluated two of these, low-molecular-weight heparin (LMWH) and recombinant hirudin (r-hirudin), in an animal (dog) model of CPB. Both compounds were found to be effective anticoagulants in these experiments. An interesting observation was the effect of these agents on 2-hour post-CPB blood loss in comparison to heparin (Fig 8). Low-molecular-weight heparin anticoagulation was associated with more postoperative bleeding than either heparin or r-hirudin. Aprotinin at 60,000 KIU/kg, as expected, reduced blood loss in the heparin group of animals but had no effect on either the r-hirudin or LMWH group blood loss.[42] The mechanism to explain these data is as yet unclear.

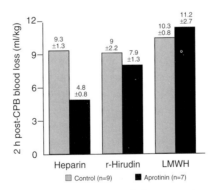

Fig 8. The effect of aprotinin treatment on 2 hour post cardiopulmonary bypass blood loss using heparin, recombinant hirudin or low molecular weight heparin (LMWH) for anticoagulation during bypass in an animal model.

SUMMARY

The mechanism of action of aprotinin, and most other drugs, is not fully understood. Our knowledge of the endogenous interactions of drugs and between drugs as related to bleeding risk is also far from complete. Drug-drug interactions need to be studied to define: (1) positive clinical effects; (2) enhanced bleeding risk (or other side effects); (3) dosage modifications needed if several drugs are used in combination; and (4) effect on laboratory assays to ensure quality of accurate information. Since most drugs have multiple sites of action and the effects of drug-drug interactions are typically not studied in preclinical trials, caution is warranted during early clinical use of a new drug.

References

1. Bick R. *Disorders of Thrombosis and Hemostasis: Clinical and Laboratory Practice*. Chicago,Ill: ASCP Press; 1992.

2. Marcum JA, Rosenberg RD. Role of endothelial cell surface heparin-like polysaccharides. *Ann N Y Acad Sci* 1989;556:81-94.

3. Ornitz DM, Herr AB, Nilsson M, Westman J, Svahn CM, Waksman G. FGF binding and FGF receptor activation by synthetic heparan-derived di- and trisaccharides. *Science* 1995;268:432-436.

4. Chan P, Mill S, Mulloy B, Kakkar V, Demoliou Mason C. Heparin inhibition of human vascular smooth muscle cell hyperplasia. *Int Angiol* 1992;11:261-267.

5. Loscalzo J, Melnick B, Handin RI. The interaction of platelet factor 4 and glycosaminoglycans. *Arch Biochem Biophys.* 1985;240:446-455.

6. Wu HF, Lundbled RL, Church FC. Neutralization of herapin activity by neutrophil lactoferrin. *Blood.* 1995;85:421-428.

7. Hoppensteadt DA, Walenga JM, Fasanella A, Jeske W, Fareed J. TFPI antigen levels in normal human volunteers after intravenous and subcutaneous administration of unfractionated heparin and a low molecular weight heparin. *Thromb Res* 1995;77:175-185.

8. Kijowski R, Hoppensteadt D, Walenga J, Borris L, Lassen MR, Fareed J. Role of tissue factor pathway inhibitor in postsurgical deep venous thrombosis (DVT) prophylaxis in patients treated with low molecular weight heparin. *Thromb Res* 1994;74:53-64.

9. Neuhaus KL, von Essen R, Tebbe U, et al. Safety observations from the pilot phase of the randomized r-Hirudin for Improvement of Thrombolysis (HIT-III) study. A study of the Arbeitsgemeinschaft Leitender Kardiologischer Krankenhausarzte (ALKK). *Circulation* 1994;90:1638-1642. Comments.

10. Antman EM. Hirudin in acute myocardial infarction: safety report from the Thrombolysis and Thrombin Inhibition in Myocardial Infarction (TIMI) 9A trial. *Circulation* 1994;90:1624-1630. Comments.

11. The Global Use of Strategies to Open Occluded Coronary Arteries (GUSTO) IIa Investigators. Randomized trial of intravenous heparin versus recombinant hirudin for acute coronary syndromes. *Circulation* 1994;90:1631-1637. Comments.

12. Walenga J, Pifarré R. Blood preservation in cardiac surgery at Loyola University Medical Center. In: Pifarré R, ed. *Anticoagulation, Hemostasis and Blood Preservation in Cardiovascular Surgery.* Philadelphia,Pa: Hanley & Belfus Inc; 1993:77-83.

13. Pifarré R, Babka R, Sullivan HJ, Montoya A, Bakhos M, El Etr A. Management of postoperative heparin rebound following cardiopulmonary bypass. *J Thorac Cardiovasc Surg* 1981;81:378-381.

14. Harker LA. Bleeding after cardiopulmonary bypass. *N Engl J Med* 1986;314:1446-1448. Editorial.

15. Bick R. Physiology and pathophysiology of hemostasis during cardiac surgery. In: Pifarré R, ed. *Blood Conservation With Aprotinin.* Philadelphia,Pa: Hanley & Belfus; 1995:199-214.

16. Lemmer JH Jr, Stanford W, Bonney SL, et al. Aprotinin for coronary bypass operations: efficacy, safety, and influence on early saphenous vein graft patency. A multicenter, randomized, double-blind, placebo-controlled study. *J Thorac Cardiovasc Surg* 1994;107:543-551.

17. Bidstrup BP, Royston D, Sapsford RN, Taylor KM. Reduction in blood loss and blood use after cardiopulmonary bypass with high dose aprotinin (Trasylol). *J Thorac Cardiovasc Surg* 1989;97:364-372.

18. Blauhut B, Gross C, Necek S, Doran J, Späth P, Lundsgaard-Anderson P. Effects of high-dose aprotinin on blood loss, platelet function, fibrinolysis, complement, and renal function after cardiopulmonary bypass. *J Thorac Cardiovasc Surg* 1991;101:958-967.

19. Fritz H, Wunderer G. Biochemistry and applications of aprotinin, the kallikrein inhibitor from bovine organs. *Arzneimittelforschung* 1983;33:479-494.

20. Espana F, Estelles A, Griffin JH, Aznar J, Gilabert J. Aprotinin (Trasylol) is a competitive inhibitor of activated protein C. *Thromb Res* 1989;56:751-756.

21. Pintigny D, Dachary-Prigent J. Aprotinin can inhibit the proteolytic activity of thrombin: a fluorescence and an enzymatic study. *Eur J Biochem* 1992;207:89-95.

22. van-den-Besselaar AM, Dirven R, Bertina RM. Tissue factor-induced coagulation can be inhibited by aprotinin (Trasylol). *Thromb Haemost* 1993;69:298-299. Letter.

23. Francis J. Effects of aprotinin on white cells and hemostasis. In: Pifarré R, ed. *Blood Conservation With Aprotinin.* Philadelphia,Pa: Hanley & Belfus; 1995:199-214.

24. Marx G, Pokar H, Reuter H, Doering V, Tilsner V. The effects of aprotinin on hemostatic function during cardiac surgery. *J Cardiothorac Vasc Anesth* 1991;5:467-474.

25. Havel M, Teufelsbauer H, Knobl P, et al. Effect of intraoperative aprotinin administration on postoperative bleeding in patients undergoing cardiopulmonary bypass operation. *J Thorac Cardiovasc Surg* 1991;101:968-972.

26. van Oeveren W, Harder M, Roozendaal K, et al Aprotinin protects platelets against the initial effect of cardiopulmonary bypass. *J Thorac Cardiovasc Surg* 1990;99:788-797.

27. Huang H, Ding W, Su Z, Zhang W. Mechanism of the preserving effect of aprotinin on platelet function and its use in cardiac surgery. *J Thorac Cardiovasc Surg* 1993;106:11-18.

28. Levy J, Pifarré R, Schaaf H, et al. A multicenter, double blind, placebo-controlled trial of aprotinin for reducing blood loss and the requirements for donor blood transfusion in patients undergoing repeat coronary artery bypass grafting. *Circulation* 1995;92:2236-2244.

29. Walenga J, Koza M, Hoppensteadt D, Sullivan H, Montoya A, Pifarré R. Fibrinolysis and antifibrinolytic activity of aprotinin in cardiac surgery. In: Pifarré R, ed. *Blood Conservation With Aprotinin.* Philadelphia, Pa: Hanley & Belfus; 1995:185-197.

30. Lu H, Soria C, Commin PL, et al. Hemostasis in patients undergoing extracorporeal circulation: the effect of aprotinin (Trasylol). *Thromb Haemost* 1991;66:633-637.

31. Orchard MA, Goodchild CS, Prentice CR, et al. Aprotinin reduces cardiopulmonary bypass-induced blood loss and inhibits fibrinolysis without influencing platelets. *Br J Haematol* 1993;85:533-541.

32. Primack C, Walenga J, Koza M, Shankey T, Pifarré R. Aprotinin modulation of platelet activation in patients undergoing cardiopulmonary bypass surgery. 1996; *Ann Thor Surg.* In press.

33. Bull B, Huse W, Brauer F, Korpeman R. Heparin therapy during extracorporeal circulation II: the use of a dose-response curve to individualize heparin and protamine dosage. *J Thorac Cardiovasc Surg* 1975;69:685-689.

34. Najman DM, Walenga JM, Fareed J, Pifarré R. Effects of aprotinin on anticoagulant monitoring: implications in cardiovascular surgery. *Ann Thorac Surg* 1993;55:662-666.

35. Young J, Kleker C, Doty O. Adequate anticoagulation during cardiopulmonary bypass determined by activated clotting time and the appearance of fibrin monomer. *Ann Thorac Surg* 1978;26:231-240.

36. de Smet AA, Joen MC, van Oeveren W, et al. Increased anticoagulation during cardiopulmonary bypass by aprotinin. *J Thorac Cardiovasc Surg* 1990;100:520-527.

37. Harder MP, Eijsman L, Roozendaal KJ, van Oeveren W, Wildevuur CR. Aprotinin reduces intraoperative and postoperative blood loss in membrane oxygenator cardiopulmonary bypass. *Ann Thorac Surg* 1991;51:936-941.

38. Cosgrove DM, Heric B, Lytle BW, et al. Aprotinin therapy for reoperative myocardial revascularization: a placebo-controlled study. *Ann Thorac Surg* 1992;54:1031-1036.

39. Royston D. High-dose aprotinin therapy: a review of the first five year's experience. *J Cardiothorac Vasc Anesth* 1992; 6:76-100.

40. Hunt BJ, Segal HC, Yacoub M. Guidelines for monitoring heparin by the activated clotting time when aprotinin is used during cardiopulmonary bypass. *J Thorac Cardiovasc Surg.* 1992;104:211-212. Letter; Comment.

41. Wang JS, Lin CY, Hung WT, Karp RB. Monitoring of heparin-induced anticoagulation with kaolin-activated clotting time in cardiac surgical patients treated with aprotinin. *Anesthesiology* 1992;77:1080-1084.

42. Terrell M, Walenga J, Koza M, Pifarré R. Efficacy of aprotinin with various anticoagulants in cardiopulmonary bypass. 1996; *Ann Thor Surg.* In press.

Index